HEALTH UNIT COORDINATOR

A Guide for Certification Review and Job Readiness

Donna J. Kuhns, CHUC

Health Unit Coordinator Instructor
Aurora Health Care
Milwaukee, Wisconsin

Patricia Noonan Rice, BA, CHUC

Association Management and Staff Development Provider
Rockford, Illinois

Linda L. Winslow, BS, CHUC

Staff Development Coordinator
Marquette General Health System
Marquette, Michigan

THOMSON

✦

DELMAR LEARNING ™

Australia   Brazil   Canada   Mexico   Singapore   Spain   United Kingdom   United States

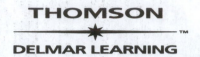

THOMSON
DELMAR LEARNING

Health Unit Coordinator: A Guide for Certification Review and Job Readiness
Donna J. Kuhns, Patricia Noonan Rice, Linda L. Winslow

Vice President,
Health Care Business Unit:
William Brottmiller

Director of Learning Solutions:
Matthew Kane

Acquisitions Editor:
Matthew Seeley

Editorial Assistant:
Megan Tarquinio

Product Manager:
Debra Flis

Marketing Director:
Jennifer McAvey

Marketing Manager:
Michele C. McTighe

Marketing Coordinator:
Andrea Eobstel

Art Director:
Jack Pendleton

Production Director:
Carolyn Miller

Content Project Manager:
Anne Sherman

Library of Congress Cataloging-in-Publication Data

Kuhns, Donna J.
  Health unit coordinator : a guide for certification review and job readiness / Donna J. Kuhns, Patricia Noonan Rice, Linda L. Winslow.
    p. cm.
  Includes bibliographical references and index.
  ISBN-13: 978-1-4180-5245-4 (alk. paper)
  ISBN-10: 1-4180-5245-0 (alk. paper)
  1. Hospital ward clerks—Examinations, questions, etc. I. Rice, Patricia (Patricia Noonan) II. Winslow, Linda L. III. Title.
  RA972.55.K845 2005 Suppl.
  362.11068—dc22

2007023878

NOTICE TO THE READER

This guide is dedicated in loving memory of Aaron Winslow. Aaron inspired all who knew him with his spirit of determination and his belief that "fun" is one of the important goals we should all strive for.

We wrote this guide to include a variety of activities because we believe that learning is fun. It is our wish that this guide prepare our readers to perform their health unit coordinator responsibilities and to attain their professional certification with the same "I can do this no matter what" spirit that Aaron demonstrated.

CONTENTS

■ *Prepare patient charts and perform clerical tasks for discharge or transfer to other units within the health facility 85* ■ *Notify appropriate departments and individuals when patients are discharged (e.g., home, expired, AMA, transferred, etc.) 85* ■ *Disassemble patient charts, put in appropriate order, and send to medical records office upon expiration or discharge 85* ■ *Schedule follow-up appointments 85* ■ *Schedule appointments for diagnostic work at other facilities 85* ■ *Follow organ procurement procedures 85* ■ *Schedule ground transportation for patients 85*

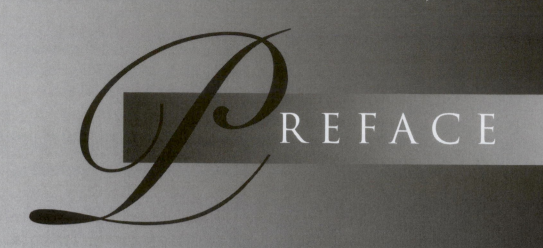

PREFACE

The health unit coordinator must continually participate in and be aware of the ongoing changes in the health care field, as well as the technology related to the health care field.

Whether you are already working as a health unit coordinator, preparing for certification, or just entering the field of health care as a novice health unit coordinator, you must have a strong understanding of medical terminology and ancillary health care departments, along with functionality within the health care system.

This book, in conjunction with the *Health Unit Coordinator: 21st Century Professional* textbook, will sharpen your skills by providing you with case scenarios and a variety of critical thinking exercises written by experienced certified health unit coordinators. This book will provide you with exercises that you can take out into the health care field to complete, which in turn will help prepare you for a successful future as a health unit coordinator. The exercises offer learners the opportunity to apply the knowledge and skills they have acquired to simulated employment scenarios. The exercises bring the textbook content to life by giving learners the chance to use theory in the context of the health unit coordinator's job responsibilities. Case scenarios are written about health unit coordinators in work situations that allow them to utilize knowledge from the key content areas of the national certification exam.

For those of you preparing to sit for the national certification exam, we applaud you for your effort and commitment and extend our best wishes. You too will find the case scenarios realistic and thought provoking. In addition to multiple-choice questions, the different types of exercises in the guide include crossword puzzles, the matching of terms to their definitions and current medical terminology on subjects that include regulatory agency guidelines, and advance directives, along with a chapter dedicated solely to computers. As in our textbook, professional development and training are also covered in this guide. The exercises can be used to expand one's knowledge of the health unit coordinator's relationship to regulatory agencies such as the Joint Commission (JC), the Health Insurance Portability and Accountability Act (HIPAA), and the Occupational Safety and Health Administration (OSHA). Exercises can be used to gain a more thorough understanding of ever-changing key issues such as case management, health care technology and electronic health records, and confidentiality.

In addition to the critical thinking exercises, many multiple-choice questions are included to give the learner practice in answering questions that are formatted like the national certification exam. Multiple-choice questions are included in each chapter and also in a set of review questions at the end of the book. This set of questions is a

50-item review that parallels the current content outline of the national certification exam. Thirty-five percent of the review questions fall under the category of transcription of orders, 47% are on the coordination of the health unit, 15% are on equipment and technical procedures, and 3% are on professional development.

Features of this book include:

- Follows the NAHUC certification exam content outline
- Scenarios covering the certification content outline, followed by questions in the multiple-choice format as found on the certification exam
- A variety of different exercises and activities to reinforce the content
- Exercises that allow you to provide answers based on experiences in your own health care facilities
- Content that is available on perforated pages, which are convenient to use
- A new, thorough approach to test-taking tips
- Inclusion of a review question set, which follows the exam content outline as listed in the National Association of Health Unit Coordinators, Inc. Candidate Handbook

Acknowledgments

We would like to thank Thomson Delmar Learning and Deb Flis for the encouragement to write this supplement to our first book, and Thomson Delmar Learning for their commitment to our first book, *Health Unit Coordinator: 21st Century Professional*.

We would also like to thank Robert Kuhns for his support and first-line editing again in this, our second book.

We appreciate all the support from our many friends and family, especially our friends in the National Association of Health Unit Coordinators who supported us and encouraged us to write this guide. And to the many health unit coordinators whose striving for professionalism has given us the strength and foresight to complete this guide, we thank you.

Reviewers

The authors and Thomson Delmar Learning acknowledge the instructors who reviewed the manuscript and provided valuable feedback.

Joyce M. Fludd
Program Coordinator
Faculty, Health Unit Coordinator Day Program
Clover Park Technical College
Lakewood, Washington

Lori J. H. Katz, CHUC, MEd
Health Unit Coordinator Instructor

Cecil Pope, AA
CHUC-Nursing Informatics Coordinator
Scott & White Memorial Hospital
Temple, Texas

Shirley Walker Powell, BA, CHUC
Education Specialist
TriHealth, Corporate Education
Cincinnati, Ohio

Lori A. Warren, MA, RN, CPC, CCP, CLNC
Medical Department Codirector
Spencerian College
Louisville, Kentucky

About the Authors

Donna J. Kuhns, CHUC, has been employed by Aurora Health Care for 30 years, during which time she has worked as a health unit coordinator, instructor, and currently as a health unit systems analyst. She coordinates and teaches new health unit coordinators and collaborates with Aurora's information technology department and many ancillary departments on application development and enhancements affecting the communication and coordination of patient activities. Donna has served as both a region representative and director of the Education Board for the National Association of Health Unit Coordinators.

Patricia Noonan Rice, BA, CHUC, of Rockford, Illinois, has worked as both a health unit coordinator and a health unit coordinator instructor. Her teaching experience includes hospital-based and community college health unit coordinator programs, staff development programs, workshops, and seminars. Currently, she owns a business that provides association management and staff development services. She is a past Accreditation Board director and Education Board director for the National Association of Health Unit Coordinators.

Linda L. Winslow, BS, CHUC, has been employed by Marquette General Health System for over 37 years, during which time she has worked as a nurse aide, a health unit coordinator, a health unit coordinator instructor, and currently as a staff development coordinator. As part of her position, she is responsible for coordinating health unit coordinator education. Linda is currently the director of the National Association of Health Unit Coordinators Education Board.

Preparation and Test-Taking Tips

Preparing to take a national certification exam or a test for a class involves just that: *preparation*. The preparation must begin well in advance of the test itself. Following are some tips that should help guide you to a successful outcome.

DAYS BEFORE THE EXAM

*A*sk instructor to specify topics that will be on the test.

*B*udget your time. Be sure you allow time to study well before the exam.

*C*areful note taking.

*D*o not cram; be sure to get at least six hours of sleep the night before the exam.

DAY OF EXAM

*E*at a good breakfast the morning of the exam.

*F*ive to ten minutes prior to the exam, arrive at the exam location.

*G*o use the restroom before entering the classroom.

*H*ave at least two sharpened pencils with you.

*I*magine yourself doing well on the test.

*J*ust clear your mind of other obligations and distractions.

*K*eep reminding yourself why the exam is important to you.

*L*et yourself concentrate totally on the task at hand.

*M*inimize discomfort—dress comfortably in layers.

*N*o skipping sample questions—they are there to help you.

*O*bey directions carefully.

*P*erform as fast as you can while still being careful and thorough—the mind works best under some pressure.

*Q*uell the urge to keep changing answers back and forth.

*R*ead all instructions, questions, and answers thoroughly.

*S*elect the closest answer even if you think it's not 100% correct.

*T*ake the easy questions first—this helps to keep your mind moving.

*U*pset stomach and fast heartbeat are usual signs of anxiety and, if mild, are normal.

*V*alue your first hunch—if you've studied and prepared, your first answer is most likely correct.

*W*atch for careless errors; double-check your work after you complete the test.

X or flag difficult questions and return to them—don't lose your momentum.

*Y*ou can guess if you have to; usually any answer is better than no answer.

*Z*ealously keep at it—never give up.

Tips for Multiple-Choice Tests

Multiple-choice questions are common on standardized tests. A multiple-choice question will have a question or incomplete statement followed by several choices from which to choose. There are usually four answer choices; one of the choices is the correct answer and the other three choices are *distracters*, or incorrect answers. The incorrect answers are called distracters because they are written to divert the test taker from the correct answer. The test taker should identify and eliminate the distracters and choose the best possible answer.

1. Try to answer the question before you look at the possible choices. If the answer you have come up with is one of the choices, mark it as the correct answer. For example:

Read the question, "Coumadin is classified as which of the following?" Try to recall the answer before you look at the choices. Perhaps you recall that coumadin is a blood thinner. Now look at the possible choices:

a. Anticonvulsant

b. Antibiotic

c. Anticoagulant

d. Analgesia

You remember that blood thinner is another term for anticoagulant, and Coumadin is a blood thinner, so you choose "c." as your answer.

2. If you're unsure of the correct answer, eliminate the distracters that are clearly wrong. For example:

Read the question, "What was the approximate first year that the health unit coordinator position was utilized in the United States?" The choices given to you are:

a. 1780

b. 1940

c. 1990

d. 1740

You may think that you can eliminate a. 1780 and d. 1740 immediately because common sense leads you to believe that these dates are way too early in U.S. history. Then you think that you can eliminate c. 1990 because you remember that your preceptor has been working for 20 years as a health unit coordinator, and that was before 1990. After eliminating the distracters, this leaves you with "b." for an answer.

3. When two of the choices are exact opposites, one of the two is often the correct answer. This may help you narrow your choices to two answers. For example:

Read the incomplete statement, "The differential blood test reports _____."

The choices given to you are:

a. various types of RBCs

b. different clotting times

c. various types of WBCs

d. all of the above

You may remember that RBCs are red blood cells and WBCs are white blood cells, so these two options are opposites; as a result, you may eliminate b and d as distracters. You might also remember that RBCs and WBCs are reported in a complete blood count, and that the white blood cells are reported in the differential. Therefore, "c." is the correct answer.

4. Information in some test questions may help you to answer other questions. It is important to try as hard as possible to finish the entire test so you will have a chance to read all of the information in all of the questions. Information from other questions may assist you once you have completed the exam and are reviewing your answers.

Resources

Canter, L. and Associates, Inc. (1989). *How to study and take tests.* (workbook)

Heidmann, C. (1983). *Test-taking skills.* (health unit coordinator class lecture)

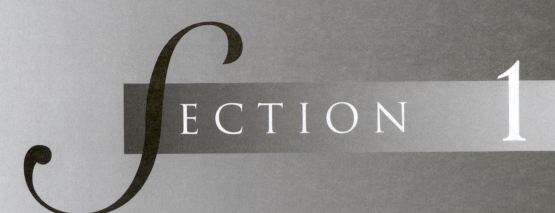

SECTION 1

Transcription of Orders

CHAPTER 1

Processing

PART A Terminology

Recommended Reading

1. Read and review Chapters 20–21 in *Health Unit Coordinator: 21st Century Professional*.

2. Read and review key terms at beginning of Chapters 14 and 23–31 in *Health Unit Coordinator: 21st Century Professional*.

Abbreviations

CHF   congestive heart failure

COPD   chronic obstructive pulmonary disease

KCL   potassium chloride

Key Terms

Arthritis   inflammation of the joints

Cholecystectomy   removal of the gallbladder

Hypertension   high blood pressure

Splenomegaly   enlarged spleen

CASE SCENARIO

Sol is the certified health unit coordinator on an orthopedic nursing unit. It is the middle of the flu season, and, since a number of health unit coordinators have called in ill, Sol has been asked to float to a medical teaching unit. On one of the charts on which she is working, she encounters some difficulty when reading through the orders; she goes to the history and physical section of the chart in an attempt to better understand what the physicians are requesting. She reads through the history and physical and notes the following:

The patient has a history of congestive heart failure, chronic obstructive pulmonary disease (COPD), hypertension, and arthritis. Past hospitalizations for splenomegaly and a cholecystectomy are also noted. The patient is allergic to penicillin and aspirin, and is currently taking atenolol BID, hydrochlorothiazide BID, Motrin Q6hr prn, and potassium chloride TID.

The patient has been using 2 liters per minute of oxygen continuously at home for the past year.

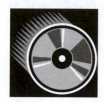

The patient has had an echocardiogram, an electrocardiogram, and a CT scan of the chest in the recent past.

After reading through the history and physical, Sol is now able to recognize some of the abbreviations she was having problems reading on the chart.

Case Scenario Questions

Based on the case scenario, define the following abbreviations.

1. QID _____

2. ASA _____

3. PCN _____

4. H & P _____

5. CHF _____

6. 02 at 2 L _____

7. COPD _____

8. CBI _____

9. DO _____

10. CMS _____

Multiple Choice Questions

1. Which selection(s) best explains an echocardiogram?
   a. Often abbreviated as "echo"
   b. An ultrasound of the heart
   c. An exam that records electrical activity of the heart
   d. Both a and b

2. *Hypertension* is best defined as:
   a. High blood sugar
   b. High blood pressure
   c. Low blood pressure
   d. Overactive

3. Which of the following are medications commonly prescribed for hypertension?
   a. Penicillin and hydrochlorothiazide
   b. Motrin and atenolol
   c. Atenolol and hydrochlorothiazide
   d. Hydrochlorothiazide and aspirin

4. *Arthritis* is defined as:
   a. Incision of the arms
   b. Inflammation of the knee
   c. Inflammation of the joints
   d. Incision of the knee

5. *Splenomegaly* is defined as:
   a. Pain around the spleen
   b. Inflammation of the spleen
   c. Removal of the spleen
   d. Enlarged spleen

6. TID is an abbreviation for which of the following?
   a. Two times a day
   b. Three times a day
   c. Four times a day
   d. Once a day

7. Which of the following best defines an electrocardiogram?
   a. An ultrasound of the heart
   b. An exam that records the electrical impulses of the heart
   c. An X-ray for the heart
   d. A heart scan

8. COPD is an abbreviation for which of the following?
   a. Congestive obstruction pulmonary disease
   b. Congestive operative pulmonary disease
   c. Chronic obstructive pulmonary diagnosis
   d. Chronic obstructive pulmonary disease

9. KCL is an approved abbreviation for which of the following?
   a. Vitamin K
   b. Vitamin K with chloride
   c. Potassium
   d. Potassium chloride

10. *Cholecystectomy* is the medical term for which of the following?
    a. Removal of the gall bladder
    b. Surgical opening of the abdomen
    c. Cutting of the gall bladder
    d. To look into the abdomen

True/False

1. "Cele" is a suffix that means tumor or hernia.
   a. True
   b. False

2. "Peri" is a prefix that means around or surrounding.
   a. True
   b. False

3. "Stomy" is a suffix that means artificial or surgical opening.
   a. True
   b. False

4. "Cide" is a suffix that means kill or destroy.
   a. True
   b. False

5. "Ren" is a prefix that means nose.
   a. True
   b. False

6. "Polio" is a word root that relates to the gray matter of the brain.
   a. True
   b. False

7. "Pyel" is a word root that means renal pelvis.
   a. True
   b. False

8. "Ambi" is a prefix that means one.
   a. True
   b. False

9. "Brady" is a prefix that means fast.
   a. True
   b. False

10. "Pseudo" is a word root that means false.
    a. True
    b. False

11. "Salping" is a prefix that means fallopian tube.
    a. True
    b. False

12. "Stomat" is a word root that means stomach.
    a. True
    b. False

13. "Myel" is a word root that means muscle.
    a. True
    b. False

14. "Inter" is a prefix that means within.
    a. True
    b. False

15. "Intra" is a prefix that means between.
    a. True
    b. False

16. "Oophor" is a word root that means ovary.
    a. True
    b. False

17. "Rrhagia" and "rrhea" are both suffixes that mean abnormal or excessive discharge.
    a. True
    b. False

18. "Sis" is a suffix that means process or condition.
    a. True
    b. False

19. "Centsis" is a suffix that means to cut.
    a. True
    b. False

20. "Malacia" is a suffix that means softening.
    a. True
    b. False

Crossword Puzzle

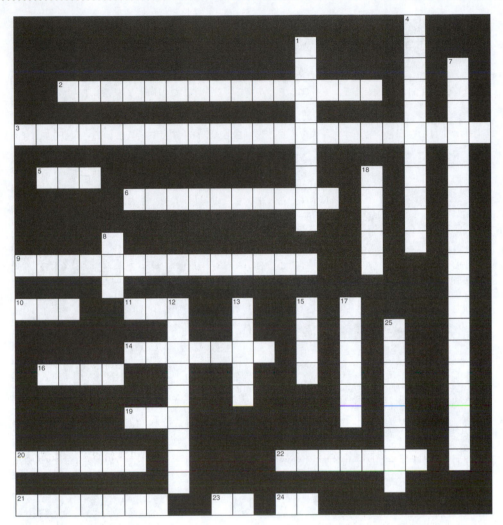

ACROSS

2. Surgical removal of the gallbladder
3. Abbreviated as CHF
5. Approved abbreviation for history and physical
6. Abbreviated as PCN
9. An ultrasound examination of the heart
10. An approved abbreviation for electrocardiogram
11. Prefix that means painful or difficult
14. Word root for fallopian tube
16. Word root that means bladder
19. Word root that means ear
20. Suffix that means development
21. Suffix that means to suture
22. Suffix that means softening
23. Suffix that means pertaining to
24. Suffix that means pertaining to

DOWN

1. Inflammation of the joints
4. Abbreviation for oxygen at 2 liters per nasal cannula
7. A medication abbreviated as HCTZ
8. Approved abbreviation for potassium chloride
12. Suffix that means hardening
13. Abnormally low, or a deficiency
15. Word root for renal pelvis
17. Prefix that means false
18. Prefix that means between
25. Puncture

■ CROSSWORD PUZZLE ANSWER

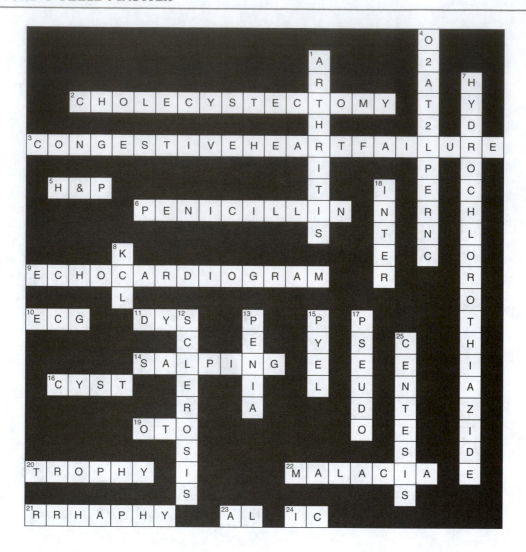

■ CASE SCENARIO ANSWERS

1. Four times a day
2. ASA is an abbreviation for aspirin.
3. PCN is an abbreviation for penicillin.
4. History and physical
5. Congestive heart failure
6. Oxygen at 2 liters
7. Chronic obstructive pulmonary disease
8. Continuous bladder irrigation
9. Doctor of osteopathy
10. Circulation, motion sensation

■ MULTIPLE CHOICE ANSWERS WITH RATIONALES

1. **d.** An echocardiogram is abbreviated as an "echo" and is an ultrasound of the heart. (page 440)
2. **b.** The prefix "hyper" means high, and "tension" refers to blood pressure. (page 337)
3. **c.** Atenolol and hydrochlorothiazide are medications that are commonly prescribed for high blood pressure. (page 515)
4. **c.** "Arthr" is the word root for joint, and "itis" is the suffix that means inflammation. (pages 339 and 344)
5. **b.** "Splen" is the word root for spleen, and "megaly" is the suffix that means enlargement. (page 345)
6. **b.** "TID" is the approved medical abbreviation for "three times a day." (page 377)
7. **b.** An electrocardiogram is the term used for the exam that records the electrical impulses of the heart. (page 440)
8. **d.** COPD is the approved medical abbreviation for chronic obstructive pulmonary disease. (Consult your medical dictionary.)
9. **d.** Potassium chloride is abbreviated as KCL. (Consult your Physician's Desk Reference.)
10. **a.** "Chole cyst" are the word roots for gall bladder, and "ectomy" is the suffix that means removal. (page 339)

■ TRUE/FALSE ANSWERS

1. **b.** False; "cele" is a *prefix* that means tumor or hernia. (page 339)
2. **a.** True (page 338)
3. **a.** True (page 345)
4. **a.** True (page 344)
5. **b.** False; "ren" is a word root that means kidney or renal. (page 343)
6. **a.** True (page 342)
7. **a.** True (page 342)
8. **b.** False; "ambi" is a prefix that means both. (page 336)
9. **b.** False; "brady" is a prefix that means slow. (page 337)
10. **a.** True (page 342)
11. **b.** False; "salping" is *word root* that means fallopian tube. (page 343)
12. **b.** False; "stomat" is a word root that means mouth. (page 343)
13. **b.** False; "myelo" is a word root that means marrow or spinal cord. (page 341)
14. **b.** False; "inter" is a prefix that means between. (page 339)
15. **b.** False; "intra" is a prefix that means within. (page 339)
16. **a.** True (page 341)
17. **a.** True (page 345)
18. **a.** True (page 345)
19. **b.** False; "centesis" is a suffix that means to puncture. (page 344)
20. **a.** True (page 345)

PART B Transcription: The Process

- ◆ Check charts for orders that need to be transcribed.

- ◆ Clarify questionable orders.

- ◆ Prioritize orders and tasks.

- ◆ Process orders according to priority.

- ◆ Enter orders on a Kardex.

- ◆ Enter orders on patient treatment plan.

- ◆ Initiate pathway protocols.

Recommended Reading

Read and review Chapters 4, 18, and 23 of *Health Unit Coordinator: 21st Century Professional*.

Key Terms

Critical pathways   information about the expected course of treatment and outcomes for a diagnostic-related group; key elements from the case management plan

Effective   successful, or achieving the desired result

Efficient   producing the desired result with a minimum use of resources, time, and effort

CASE SCENARIO

Hoang is a certified health unit coordinator on a general medical unit. Hoang is reporting for duty at the beginning of his shift. The health unit coordinator working the shift before Hoang was pulled away from the unit and sent to another department to work. Hoang is beginning his shift facing several unfinished orders and tasks in addition to his routine duties. Hoang knows he must first prioritize the pending tasks and organize his work for the day. Hoang has a tool he calls his "brainboard," which is a "to-do" list he uses to stay organized. As Hoang begins to plan his day, he always keeps patient safety as his main goal and focus. He also keeps in mind the length of time it will take to complete each task. Hoang knows he can

(continued)

perform some of the smaller tasks quickly; he will also group tasks that can be performed together. Hoang is experienced at multi-tasking, or doing several things at once. Hoang is an effective and efficient worker, and he never loses sight of the fact that safety and accuracy are most important.

This is what Hoang encounters as he begins his shift:

1. Patient charges must be entered into the computer before the end of the shift.
2. Admission charts must be set up for the next shift.
3. Pages of laboratory results from the fax printer must be filed in the patient's chart.
4. The fax printer is out of paper.
5. A nurse is calling out for a stat respiratory treatment in her patient's room.
6. A family member is at the desk requesting to speak with the hospital chaplain.
7. A voice mail from Social Service has been left, requesting that copies be made for a patient who is going to an extended-care facility tomorrow.
8. A physician has flagged two charts with stat orders.
9. A specimen to be sent to the lab is sitting on the desk and is marked "stat."
10. Charts have to be checked for new orders.
11. An e-mail has been sent from the health unit coordinator educator, reminding Hoang about a continuing education class at lunchtime today.

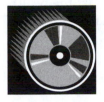

Case Scenario Questions

1. List the 11 tasks in the order in which you think Hoang should complete them. Explain why you chose the order you did.

   _____

   _____

   _____

   _____

   _____

   _____

   _____

   _____

   _____

   _____

   _____

   _____

Multiple Choice Questions

1. *Flagging* is best described as:
   a. The process of identifying the patient's physician on the chart
   b. The process of identifying the patient's next of kin on the chart
   c. The process of drawing attention to new physician orders in the chart
   d. The process of drawing attention to patient allergies in the chart

2. It is important for the health unit coordinator to recognize orders that need to be transcribed because:
   a. Orders must be transcribed in a timely fashion
   b. The Patients' Bill of Rights mandates that orders must be transcribed within 30 minutes
   c. The health unit coordinator must read the new orders to the patient
   d. None of the above

3. To recognize orders that need transcribing, the health unit coordinator may look for:
   a. A phone message from the physician's office stating that there are new orders
   b. An incident report stating that new orders were missed
   c. A notation in the physician's progress notes stating that there are new orders
   d. The absence of sign-off information

4. Which of the following may be used for flagging?
   a. A brightly colored marker or card inserted in the chart
   b. A light system outside the patient's room
   c. Both a and b
   d. None of the above

5. Which of the following is a true statement about health unit coordinators and order clarification?
   a. A novice health unit coordinator is not expected to recognize any orders that need clarification.
   b. A health unit coordinator must follow the employer's protocol for order clarification.
   c. A health unit coordinator may fill in missing components on routine physician orders to save time instead of seeking clarification.
   d. A health unit coordinator will always be the designated staff person to clarify physician orders.

6. Order clarification always requires communication with:
   a. The nurse
   b. The physician
   c. The health unit coordinator
   d. The patient

7. Which of the following is a tool that the health unit coordinator may use to organize tasks that need to be completed?
   a. An activity sheet
   b. A sign-in-and-out sheet
   c. A Kardex
   d. A patient treatment plan

8. What is the main factor to consider when organizing tasks in order of importance?
   a. Length of time to complete task
   b. Which tasks can be grouped together
   c. The patient's schedule
   d. Patient safety

9. Which of the following is the correct order for transcribing orders?
   a. Routine, asap, stat
   b. Stat, routine, asap
   c. Asap, stat, routine
   d. Stat, asap, routine

10. Which of the following statements about the Kardex is false?
    a. It does not change.
    b. It may be in paper or electronic form.
    c. Normally, erasures and deletions are allowed.
    d. It is a profile of all current physician orders for a patient.

CRITICAL THINKING EXERCISE

Kardex

Take this worksheet to your internship or work site to answer the following questions. Obtain permission from your work site to review a Kardex.

1. Describe the Kardex you viewed. Was it paper or electronic? If it was a paper copy, where was it filed? If it was electronic, where was it viewed?

   _____

   _____

   _____

2. List at least five examples of patient personal data found on the Kardex.

   _____

   _____

   _____

3. List the section headings found on the Kardex. For each heading, list an example of an order.

   _____

   _____

   _____

4. List the dates of the oldest and the most recent orders on the Kardex.

   _____

   _____

   _____

CRITICAL THINKING EXERCISE

Pathway Protocol

Case management is defined in Health Unit Coordinator: 21st Century Professional *as a management system in which the case manager reviews patient care and changes systems to reflect the best possible treatment with the best possible outcomes.*

For more information about case management and pathways, read the following excerpt from DeLaune and Ladner's *Fundamentals of Nursing: Standards and Practice*, 2nd edition (Clifton Park, NY: Delmar):

> A methodology for organizing client care through an episode of illness so that specific clinical and financial outcomes are achieved within an allotted time frame. . . . The outcome of this process is a diagnostic-related group (DRG) specific case management plan that contains daily assessment documentation, care plan, outcome oriented multidisciplinary interventions, teaching and discharge planning. At admission, the nurse case manager and admitting practitioner individualize the case management plan (called a critical pathway) to meet the client's specific needs. A critical pathway is an abbreviated summary of key elements from the case management plan. The pathway is used by all health care providers as a monitoring and documentation tool to ensure that interventions are performed on time and that client outcomes are achieved on time. (pp. 516–517)

> The advantages of case management are that it makes efficient use of time and increases the quality of care, with the expected outcomes identified on the plan. It also promotes collaboration, communication, and teamwork, which work to the advantage of the client and the facility, with discharge occurring in a timely manner.

Take this worksheet to your internship or work site to answer the following questions. Obtain permission from your work site to review a patient care plan or pathway.

1. List the diagnosis for the care plan/pathway you viewed.

   _____

   _____

   _____

2. List one of the patient goals for the care plan/pathway you viewed.

   _____

   _____

   _____

3. List one action to help the patient achieve the goal.

   _____

   _____

   _____

4. Ask the unit coordinator at the work site who initiates the care plan/pathway. Record the answer.

   _____

   _____

   _____

5. Ask the unit coordinator at the work site about his or her interaction with the care plan/pathway. Record the answer.

   _____

   _____

   _____

■ CASE SCENARIO ANSWERS

1. A nurse is calling out for a stat respiratory treatment in her patient's room.
2. A physician has flagged two charts with stat orders.
3. A family member is at the desk requesting to speak with the hospital chaplain.
4. A specimen to be sent to the lab is sitting on the desk and is marked "stat."
5. The fax printer is out of paper.
6. Charts have to be checked for new orders.
7. Pages of laboratory results from the fax printer must be filed in the patient's chart.
8. An email has been sent from the health unit coordinator educator, reminding Hoang about a continuing education class at lunchtime today.
9. A voice mail from Social Service has been left, requesting that copies be made for a patient who is going to an extended-care facility tomorrow.
10. Patient charges must be entered into the computer before the end of the shift.
11. Admission charts must be set up for the next shift.

The unit coordinator may decide to first respond to the nurse's stat request for a respiratory treatment and page the respiratory therapist. While the unit coordinator is waiting for the response to the page to respiratory, he can quickly review the stat orders. Almost simultaneously, he can assure the patient's family that he will contact the chaplain. Next, he may decide to get the stat specimen to the lab. He can also quickly load the fax printer with paper to ensure that laboratory results and other information are being received as soon as they are transmitted. Once these tasks are out of the way, he will likely return to the stat orders. When that is complete, he may check the charts for new orders and, at the same time, file lab results in the charts. He will then attend his lunchtime meeting. After the meeting, he can make sure copies are made for the extended care facility transfer, enter charges, and set up admission charts for the next shifts. All the while, he will utilize his "to-do" list to keep his tasks organized.

■ MULTIPLE CHOICE ANSWERS WITH RATIONALES

1. **c.** *Flagging* is best described as the process of drawing attention to new physician orders in the chart. (page 390)
2. **a.** It is important for the health unit coordinator to recognize orders that need to be transcribed because orders must be transcribed in a timely fashion. (page 390)
3. **d.** To recognize orders that need transcribing, the health unit coordinator may look for the absence of sign-off information. (page 391)
4. **c.** A brightly colored marker or card inserted in the chart or a light system outside the patient's room may be used for flagging. (page 390)
5. **b.** A health unit coordinator must follow the employer's protocol for order clarification. (page 392)
6. **b.** Order clarification always requires communication with the physician. (page 392)
7. **a.** The health unit coordinator may use an activity sheet to organize tasks that need to be completed. (page 305)
8. **d.** Patient safety is the main factor to consider when organizing tasks in order of importance. (page 305)
9. **d.** Stat, asap, routine is the correct order for transcribing orders. (page 393)
10. **a.** The statement "It does not change" is false with regard to the Kardex. (page 398)

PART C Transcribing Laboratory, Diagnostic Exam, Nutrition, and Therapy

◆ Schedule diagnostic tests and procedures.

◆ Initiate and follow test preparation procedures.

◆ Identify orders specific to women.

◆ List common terminology for a labor and delivery unit.

Recommended Reading

Read and review Chapters 20, 21, 24, 25, 26, 29, and 30 of *Health Unit Coordinator: 21st Century Professional*.

Abbreviations

FHT   fetal heart tones

GC   gonorrhea

NST   non-stress test

PID   pelvic inflammatory disease

PKU   phenylketonuria

Key Terms

Capillary   a minute blood vessel that connects the ends of the smallest arteries with the beginnings of the smallest veins

Cesarean   term used when a baby is delivered through a surgical abdominal incision; also known as a C-section

Chlamydia   sexually transmitted disease

Cholelithasis   gallstone in the bile duct

Cord blood   refers to the umbilical cord (in this chapter)

Gravida   refers to the number of times a woman has been pregnant

Hepatosplenomegaly   enlarged liver and spleen

Hysterectomy   surgical removal of the uterus

Laparotomy   surgical exploratory procedure that opens the abdomen

Menorrhagia   abnormally excessive menstrual flow

Peritoneal   a membrane that lines the walls of an abdominal cavity and folds into the viscera; relating to the peritoneum

Phenylketonuria   a rare hereditary condition that can cause mental retardation if not treated

Pitocin   medication used to start or improve uterine contractions

Rubella   another name for German measles

Salpingo-oophorectomy   surgical removal of the uterus, fallopian tubes, and ovaries

CASE SCENARIO 1

Margaret is an excellent health unit coordinator who has been certified for several years. She has been asked to assist in the development of a lesson plan for new health unit coordinators regarding her facility's ancillary departments. Having worked as a health unit coordinator for 20 years, she is quite excited about this opportunity. Margaret knows that ancillary departments are very different from support departments, because the ancillary departments assist in diagnosing and treating the patient whereas support departments work more with the staff and patients to provide assistance. Margaret realizes that a good health unit coordinator must be familiar with which tests are ordered from each department. She is also aware that with lab tests, some panels may include some of the same tests. If the health unit coordinator has a good understanding of the tests, she will be able to process the requests in a more timely and efficient manner. Margaret first thinks of the most common ancillary departments, such as cardiology, radiology, and the laboratory. Then she lists the other diagnostic ancillary departments and thinks about the common tests she's ordered from them. Her list looks like this:

Cardiology

    ECG/EKG

    Echocardiogram

    Holter monitor

Digestive disorders, or the gastrointestinal (GI) department

    Bronchoscopy

    Colonoscopy

    Gastroscopy

    Proctoscopy

Pulmonary medicine, which includes respiratory therapy

    ABG stat

    CPT Q4hr534

    Induced sputum for cytology 536

    IPPB q4hr 534

    O2 at 2L/per nc 532

    PFTs 536

    Pulse Ox Q6hr 536

    IS POD1 534

    CPAP 535

Physical medicine and rehabilitation

    Hydrotherapy everyday

    OT eval for ADLs

    Crutch Walking BID NWB

    TENs

    EMG

    Video esophogram for swallowing eval

As Margaret continues to think about the ancillary departments, she decides that she should list the divisions for two large departments: laboratory and radiology. The laboratory at this facility has the following divisions:

    Blood bank

    Chemistry

    Coagulation

    Cytology

    Hematology

    Histology

    Microbiology

    Urinalysis

The radiology department is divided into the following divisions:

    Angiography

    Computerized tomography

    Diagnostic X-ray

    Magnetic resonance imaging

    Mammography

    Nuclear medicine

    Ultrasound

Case Scenario 1 Questions

1. Which of the following is the ancillary department that performs a colonoscopy?
   a. Chemistry
   b. Digestive disorders
   c. Ultrasound
   d. Urinalysis

2. Which of the following is the ancillary department that assists a patient with intermittent positive pressure breathing (IPPB)?
   a. Cardiology
   b. Diagnostic X-ray
   c. Physical medicine
   d. Respiratory therapy

3. Which of the following is the ancillary department that may have as many as eight different divisions?
   a. Digestive disorders
   b. Laboratory
   c. Physical medicine and rehabilitation
   d. Radiology

4. Which of the following is the ancillary department that assists the patient with activities of daily living?
   a. Cardiology
   b. Digestive disorders
   c. Physical medicine and rehabilitation
   d. Pulmonary medicine

5. Which of the following best defines ancillary departments?
   a. Departments that diagnose and treat patients
   b. The digestive disorders department
   c. Departments that are divided into different divisions
   d. Departments that support the personnel treating patients

6. Which of the following is the ancillary department that is also known as diagnostic imaging?
   a. Cardiology
   b. Digestive disorders
   c. Laboratory
   d. Radiology

7. Which of the following is the ancillary department that performs continuous positive airway pressure (CPAP)?

   a. Cardiology

   b. Physical medicine and rehabilitation

   c. Pulmonary

   d. Radiology

8. To schedule an echocardiogram, the health unit coordinator needs to contact which ancillary department?

   a. Cardiology

   b. Digestive disorders

   c. Pulmonary medicine

   d. Radiology

9. Which of the following is the ancillary department that performs an electromyogram?

   a. Cardiology

   b. Digestive disorders

   c. Physical medicine and rehabilitation

   d. Pulmonary medicine

10. To schedule a bronchoscopy, the health unit coordinator needs to contact which ancillary department?

    a. Digestive disorders

    b. Pulmonary medicine

    c. Physical medicine and rehabilitation

    d. Radiology

Additional Questions: Ancillary Department Exams

1. TIBC is the abbreviation for which of the following?
   a. Total iron binding capacity
   b. Timed iron binding capacity
   c. Total iron binding capillary
   d. Total iron basic capacity

2. Which tests are found in an electrolyte panel?
   a. CO_2, Cl, Na, and K
   b. Cholesterol, chloride, calcium, potassium
   c. Carbon dioxide, chloride, sodium, potassium
   d. a and c

3. Which of the following is a reason that a uric acid test is drawn?
   a. To diagnose renal failure
   b. To diagnose gout
   c. To measure liver function
   d. To evaluate for bone and liver failure

4. Which of the following is a reason that a cholesterol level is drawn?
   a. To measure liver function
   b. To study kidney function
   c. To measure the release of an enzyme
   d. a and c

5. HgbA1C is an abbreviation for which of the following?
   a. Hemoglobin ace inhibitor
   b. Hemoglobin bicarbonate
   c. Hemoglobin isolator
   d. Glycosylated hemoglobin

6. Ca is an abbreviation for which of the following?
   a. Carbon monoxide
   b. Calcium
   c. Cardiac enzyme
   d. Cortisol

7. Which of the following best defines autologous blood?
   a. Blood from a disease-free donor
   b. Another term for whole blood
   c. Blood from a local blood center
   d. A patient's own blood

8. What are the four blood types?
   a. A, B, C, and D
   b. A, B, C, and O
   c. A, B, AB, and O
   d. A, B, A positive, and A negative

9. BUN is an abbreviation for which of the following?
   a. Blood, urine, and nitrogen
   b. Blood, urea, and nitrogen
   c. Blood, urine, and sodium
   d. Blood, urea, and nickel

10. HbsAG is an abbreviation for which of the following?
    a. Hepatitis A and B antigen
    b. Hepatitis B antibody and antigen
    c. Hepatitis B surface antigen
    d. Hepatitis A and B antibody and antigen

11. From which department would you order a KUB?
    a. Cardiology
    b. Digestive disorders
    c. Radiology
    d. Physical medicine and rehabilitation

12. OCG is an abbreviation for which of the following?
    a. Oral cystogram
    b. Gall bladder x-ray
    c. Oral cholecystogram
    d. B and C

13. Which of the following are the components of a BMP?
    a. CO_2, CL, Creat, glucose, Ca, BUN, K, Na, Anion gap
    b. CL, Creat, glucose, Ca, BUN, K, Na, Anion gap
    c. CO_2, CL, Creat, glucose, Ca, BUN, K, Na, triglycerides, Anion gap
    d. CO_2, CL, Creat, glucose, Ca, BUN, K, Na, Mg, Anion gap

14. Which of the following are the components of a renal function panel?
    a. Albumin, BUN, Cl, phosphorus, Ca, Creat, CO_2, K, glucose,
    b. Albumin, BUN, Cl, phosphorus, Ca, Creat, CO_2, K, glucose, Na
    c. Albumin, ALT, BUN, Cl, phosphorus, Ca, Creat, CO_2, K, glucose,
    d. Albumin, BUN, Cl, Hct, phosphorus, Ca, Creat, CO_2, K, glucose, Na

15. HDL is an abbreviation for which of the following?
    a. High-density lipids
    b. High-defined leukocytes
    c. High-density leukocytes
    d. High-density lipoprotein

16. Which of the following best defines isoenzymes?
    a. Determine the variations in the enzymes responsible for an elevation in enzymes such as LDH
    b. Determine the variations in the enzymes responsible for an elevation in enzymes such as CK
    c. Determine the variations in the enzymes responsible for an elevation in enzymes such as CPK
    d. All of the above

17. Which of the following is a lab panel that consists of Hct, Hgb, WBC, RBC, and Diff?
    a. Hepatic function panel
    b. Complete blood count
    c. Comprehensive metabolic panel
    d. Renal function panel

18. Which ancillary department performs a DSA?
    a. Angiography
    b. Computerized tomography
    c. Nuclear medicine
    d. Ultrasound

19. EGD is an abbreviation for which of the following?
    a. Echo esophagoduogram
    b. Endoscopic gastroduodenoscopy
    c. Esophagastroduodenoscopy
    d. Esophagogastroduodenoscopy

20. Which ancillary department performs a liver/spleen scan?
    a. Computerized tomography
    b. Magnetic resonance imaging
    c. Nuclear medicine
    d. Ultrasound

21. Which ancillary department uses small amounts of radioactive materials, which are introduced to the patient intravenously?
    a. Dx X-ray
    b. Magnetic resonance imaging
    c. Nuclear medicine
    d. Ultrasound

22. BAER is an abbreviation for which of the following?
    a. Brain and auditory evoked request
    b. Brainstem auditory evoked response
    c. Brain and auditory evoked response
    d. Brainstem auditory evoked request

23. EEG is an abbreviation for which of the following?

    a. Electrocardiogram

    b. Echocardiogram

    c. Echoencephalogram

    d. Electroencephalogram

24. Which ancillary department performs an ERCP?

    a. Digestive disorders

    b. Dx X-ray

c. Nuclear medicine

d. Ultrasound

25. Which of the following is the abbreviation for a lower gastrointestinal X-ray?

    a. GB

    b. BaE

    c. IVP

    d. KUB

$\mathcal{C}$ ASE SCENARIO 2

Margaret, a certified health unit coordinator, thinks about a scenario for a typical day that she can use in class. She starts her scheduled shift at 3:00 P.M. Usually, around 10 people are admitted to the medical unit each day; if she is lucky, the charts are put together and the orders have been written and completed. Charts with orders are often waiting to be transcribed, including a "CBC in am times 4 days." From this, Margaret would know to enter the order into the computer for a complete blood count (CBC) for 7:00 A.M. over the next four days. Margaret would also enter the order information in the computer so it can be viewed on the electronic Kardex by the nursing staff. Because of her many years on the job, Margaret has a habit of sending test requests to the department before she enters things in the Kardex.

Another chart may include a diagnostic exam order for a CT scan of the abdomen. Margaret enters the test request into the computer. Margaret also processes the preparation orders for the CT scan so it can be done in the morning. A verification of the CT scan set for the following day is sent to the nursing unit from the CT department via computer, along with time information, so the nursing unit can have the patient prepped and ready by the designated time. Margaret enters that time on the Kardex. Like CT scans, ultrasounds are also common tests that require the patient to be prepped ahead of time.

Other orders written later in the day by a physician may include diet and therapy orders. For example, a diet change that can occur later in the day may be "advance diet to NAS, Lo Chol" for a patient who was previously on a DAT. Other diet changes may be needed to prepare patients for the following day's procedures, such as a "cl liq" or NPO. These are the diets that Margaret would watch for, knowing they need to be sent to the diet office as soon as possible.

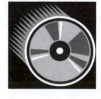

Therapy orders are also written to prepare patients for discharge during the next few days. Some of the common therapy orders Margaret sees are "Crutch walking with NWB" and "OT for ADLs." Arterial blood gases are another common order that Margaret often sees on the second shift for patients who may not be breathing very well.

Case Scenario 2 Questions

Fill in the blank with the correct word.

1. The _____ department performs tests to determine chemical changes in body fluids.
   a. Chemistry
   b. Serology
   c. Microbiology
   d. Collection

2. _____ specimens are the most common specimens collected.
   a. Urine
   b. Tissue
   c. Blood
   d. Secretion

3. The use of high-frequency sound to image internal structures is the procedure used in _____.
   a. a CT scan
   b. an MRI
   c. a PET
   d. an ultrasound

4. The abbreviation _____ is used to order meals for a patient who has been diagnosed with diabetes.
   a. DD
   b. DAD
   c. ADA
   d. ADD

5. The term "_____ diet" is given to a balanced, nutritional diet with no restrictions.
   a. regular
   b. general
   c. a and b
   d. none of the above

6. _____ is the abbreviation for "diet as tolerated."
   a. DAT
   b. AT
   c. ADV
   d. All of the above

7. _____ orders remain in place until orders are written to change or discontinue them.
   a. Elective
   b. Emergency
   c. Regular
   d. Standing

8. _____ therapy helps people regain and develop skills that are important for self-care and self-sufficiency.
   a. Speech
   b. Recreational
   c. Occupational
   d. All of the above

9. _____ is ordered to help restore motion and aid in recovery for patients.
   a. OT
   b. CR
   c. PT
   d. RT

10. Arterial blood gases (ABGs) are tests that measure the concentration of _____ and carbon dioxide in the blood.
    a. electrolytes
    b. hydrogen
    c. oxygen
    d. hemoglobin

11. "Crutch walking" with no weight bearing would be abbreviated as _____.
    a. CWN
    b. CNW
    c. NWB
    d. BNW

12. ADL is the abbreviation for "_____ of daily living."
    a. activities
    b. action
    c. active
    d. artificial

13. NPO is the abbreviation for "nothing _____."
    a. by mouth
    b. per os
    c. for the day
    d. a and b

14. Test preps should be followed for numerous _____ and CT scans.
   a. lab tests
   b. therapies
   c. ultrasounds
   d. all of the above

15. A clear liquid diet is often written as "_____ liq."
   a. C
   b. Cl
   c. Cle
   d. Free

CASE SCENARIO 3

Laura, a certified health unit coordinator, is excited and a little nervous about her upcoming interview. The health care facility where Laura works is opening a new Women's Health Center. In the Women's Health Center will be a brand new Labor and Delivery Unit and a Postpartum Unit; these will be referred to the Family Unit and the Women's Surgical Unit, respectively. There will be many other outpatient services as well, including acupuncture, aromatherapy, massage, education, nutrition, and diet counseling. Other specific amenities include an outside healing garden, fertility services, osteoporosis screening, and cancer screening and treatment. Laura would really like to be transferred to the new Women's Health Center. She has floated a few times to the small women's health unit that is currently located within her facility; she recalls that most lab work included the usual CBC, Lytes, U/A, and so forth. However, she also recalls ordering more total bilirubins, chlamydia, rubella, and syphilis tests, along with cord blood tests and capillary blood gases, on that unit. In preparation for the interview, Laura retrieves the notes that she studied while preparing for her certification exam, which she passed with 98% accuracy. The medical terms and abbreviations are listed at the beginning of this chapter.

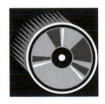

Case Scenario 3 Questions

Define the following abbreviations.

1. PID _____

2. GC _____

3. FHT _____

4. PKU _____

5. NST _____

Match the term in Column I with the correct definition in Column II.

Column I

_____ 1. Phenylketonuria

_____ 2. Cesarean

_____ 3. Cholelithasis

_____ 4. Gravida

_____ 5. Hysterectomy

_____ 6. Peritoneal

_____ 7. Capillary

_____ 8. Chlamydi

_____ 9. Cord blood

_____ 10. Hepatosplenomegaly

_____ 11. Laparotomy

_____ 12. Pitocin

_____ 13. Menorrhagia

_____ 14. Rubella

_____ 15. Salpingo-oophorectomy

Column II

a. Surgical removal of the uterus, fallopian tubes, and ovaries

b. A minute blood vessel that connects the ends of the smallest arteries with the beginnings of the smallest veins

c. Term used when a baby is delivered through a surgical abdominal incision; also known as a C-section

d. Sexually transmitted disease

e. Gallstone in bile duct

f. Another name for German measles

g. Medication used to start or improve uterine contractions

h. A rare hereditary condition that can cause mental retardation if not treated

i. A membrane that lines the walls of an abdominal cavity and folds into the viscera; relating to the peritoneum

j. Abnormally excessive menstrual flow

k. Surgical exploratory procedure that opens the abdomen

l. Surgical removal of the uterus

m. Enlarged liver and spleen

n. Refers to the number of times a woman has been pregnant

o. Refers to the umbilical cord

CRITICAL THINKING EXERCISE

Rehabilitation Services

1. List the rehabilitation services that are available in your area. Check the yellow pages and the Internet for available services.

   _____

   _____

   _____

   a. Call three different places and ask them what occupational therapy services they provide.

   _____

   _____

   _____

   b. Call three different places and ask them what physical therapy services they provide.

   _____

   _____

   _____

   If possible, visit one of the places you called. What does the area look like? Is there a marketing brochure? If so, does it explain the services offered? What are the job titles of the employed staff?

■ CASE SCENARIO 1 ANSWERS
WITH RATIONALES

1. **b.** Digestive disorders or GI departments perform colonoscopies. (page 87)

2. **d.** Respiratory therapy assists patients with IPPB. (page 534)

3. **b.** The laboratory is usually divided into at least eight different divisions. (page 89)

4. **c.** Occupational therapy is a division of physical medicine and rehabilitation. (page 539)

5. **a.** Ancillary departments are departments that diagnose and treat patients. (page 86)

6. **d.** Diagnostic imaging is another name for radiology. (page 90)

7. **c.** The pulmonary department performs CPAP. (page 536)

8. **a.** An echocardiogram is requested by the cardiology department. (page 86)

9. **c.** The physical medicine and rehabilitation department performs electromyograms. (page 539)

10. **a.** The digestive disorders or GI departments perform a bronchoscopy. (page 87)

■ ADDITIONAL QUESTIONS: ANCILLARY
DEPARTMENT EXAMS ANSWERS
WITH RATIONALES

1. **a.** TIBC stands for total iron binding capacity. (page 420)

2. **d.** Carbon dioxide (CO_2), chloride (Cl), sodium (Na), and potassium(K) make up an electrolyte panel. (page 421)

3. **b.** A uric acid test is one of the tests drawn to diagnose gout. (page 420)

4. **a.** A cholesterol level test is one of the tests drawn to measure liver function. (page 419)

5. **d.** Glycosylated hemoglobin is abbreviated as HgbA1C. (page 419)

6. **b.** Calcium is abbreviated as Ca. (page 419)

7. **d.** Autologous blood is a patient's own blood. (page 425)

8. **c.** A, B, AB, and O are the four blood types. (page 424)

9. **b.** Blood, urea, nitrogen is abbreviated as BUN. (page 419)

10. **c.** Hepatitis B surface antigen is abbreviated as HbsAG. (page 417)

11. **c.** Radiology would take an X-ray of the kidneys, ureter, and bladder, or KUB. (page 444)

12. **d.** A gall bladder X-ray—otherwise known as an oral cholecystogram—is abbreviated as OCG. (page 444)

13. **a.** CO_2, CL, Creat, glucose, Ca, BUN, K, Na, and anion gap are components of a basic metabolic panel (BMP). (page 421)

14. **b.** The components of a renal function panel include albumin, BUN, Cl, phosphorus, Ca, Creat, CO_2, K, glucose, and Na. (page 421)

15. **d.** High-density lipoprotein is abbreviated as HDL. (page 419)

16. **d.** Isoenzymes determine the variations responsible for an elevation in enzymes such as LDH, CK, and CPK. (page 420)

17. **b.** Some of the components in a complete blood count are Hct, Hgb, WBC, RBCs, and the differential panel. (page 421)

18. **a.** An angiography department would perform a DSA. (page 442)

19. **d.** EGD is the abbreviation for an esophagogastroduodenoscopy. (page 450)

20. **c.** A liver/spleen scan is performed by the nuclear medicine department. (page 446)

21. **c.** Nuclear medicine uses small amounts of radioactive materials to enhance images of a scan. (page 446)

22. **c.** BAER is the abbreviation for a brainstem auditory evoked response. (page 452)

23. **d.** EEG is the abbreviation for an electroencephalogram. (page 452)

24. **a.** An ERCP is performed in the digestive disorders department (page 450)

25. **b.** A barium enema (BaE) is another name for a lower gastrointestinal X-ray. (page 444)

■ CASE SCENARIO 2 ANSWERS WITH RATIONALES

1. **a.** The chemistry department performs tests to determine chemical changes in body fluids. (page 418)

2. **c.** Blood specimens are the most common specimens collected. (page 410)

3. **d.** An ultrasound is a procedure that uses high-frequency sound to image internal structures. (page 447)

4. **c.** ADA is the abbreviation used in diets for patients with diabetes. (page 462)

5. **c.** Both "general" and "regular" can refer to diets ordered for patients with no dietary restrictions. (page 459)

6. **a.** DAT is an approved abbreviation for "diet as tolerated." (page 459)

7. **d.** Orders that remain in place until changed or discontinued are known as standing orders. (page 468)

8. **c.** Occupational therapy helps people regain and develop skills. (page 539)

9. **c.** Physical therapy (PT) helps to restore motion and aid in recovery for patients. (page 538)

10. **c.** ABGs are ordered to measure the concentration of oxygen and carbon dioxide in the blood. (page 536)

11. **c.** NWB is the abbreviation for "no weight bearing." (page 538)

12. **a.** ADL is the abbreviation for "activities of daily living." (page 539)

13. **d.** NPO stands for "nothing per os" or "nothing by mouth." (page 376)

14. **c.** Patients often need to be prepped for ultrasounds and CT scans. (page 448)

15. **b.** Cl liq is an approved abbreviation for "clear liquids." (page 457)

■ CASE SCENARIO 3 ANSWERS WITH RATIONALES

Abbreviation answers:

1. PID: pelvic inflammatory disease
2. GC: gonorrhea
3. FHT: fetal heart tone
4. PKU: phenylketonuria
5. NST: non-stress test

Matched definitions answers:

1. **b.** Phenylketonuria is a rare hereditary condition that can cause mental retardation if not treated.

2. **c.** Cesarean is the term used when a baby is delivered through a surgical abdominal incision; also known as a C-section.

3. **e.** Cholelithasis is a gallstone in the bile duct.

4. **n.** Gravida refers to the number of times a woman has been pregnant.

5. **l.** A hysterectomy is the surgical removal of the uterus.

6. **i.** Peritoneal is a membrane that lines the walls of an abdominal cavity and folds into the viscera; relating to the peritoneum.

7. **b.** Capillary refers to a minute blood vessel that connects the ends of the smallest arteries with the beginnings of the smallest veins.

8. **d.** Chlamydia is a sexually transmitted disease.

9. **o.** Cord blood refers to the umbilical cord.

10. **m.** Hepatosplenomegaly is an enlarged liver and spleen.

11. **k.** Laparotomy refers to a surgical exploratory procedure that opens the abdomen.

12. **g.** Pitocin is a medication used to start or improve uterine contractions.

13. **j.** Menorrhagia refers to an abnormally excessive menstrual flow.

14. **f.** Rubella is another name for German measles.

15. **a.** Salpingo-oophorectomy is the surgical removal of the uterus, fallopian tubes, and ovaries.

PART D Transcribing Medications and Intravenous Therapy Orders

◆ Enter orders into a medication administration record.

◆ Enter patient charges.

Recommended Reading

1. Read and review Chapter 28 in *Health Unit Coordinator: 21st Century Professional*.

2. Read and review the key terms at beginning of Chapter 28 in Health *Unit Coordinator: 21st Century Professional*.

Abbreviation

KCL   potassium chloride

Key Terms

Antihyperlipidemics   class of drugs used to reduce blood lipids or fats; fatty-acid medications.

Controlled substances   a dangerous drug that has no recognized medical use; known as a Schedule I drug

Corticosteroids   synthetic drug used to treat a variety of conditions

Total parenteral nutrition   the practice of feeding a person by bypassing the gastrointestinal system and infusing nutrients directly into the bloodstream

CASE SCENARIO

Courtney is a newly hired certified health unit coordinator. After she received a certificate in health unit coordinating, she took an extended vacation before applying for jobs and starting her career. Now that she is working, she is experiencing some difficulty transcribing medications orders. She remembers that all medication orders have four component parts—the name of the medication, the dose, the route, and the frequency.

Preprinted orders make reading the orders easier, but Courtney believes that reviewing certain points of medication transcription will allow her to be more accurate and confident when transcribing medications orders.

She remembers that medication names are either listed as the chemical name, generic name, or brand name. In addition, she notices that the doses used at her facility are mostly metric doses—a more common, modern measurement of weights. Courtney makes herself a list for quick reference, as shown here:

Weights	Fluids
1 gram = 1000 milligrams	1 liter = 1000 milliliters
1 milligram = 1000 micrograms	1 milliliter = 1 cubic centimeter
1 gram = 1 milliliter	
1 kilogram = 1 liter	
1 pound = 16 ounces	

Courtney does not see many intramuscular (IM) orders; she sees mostly oral (po) medications. It is the patient-controlled analgesia (PCA) orders and the vascular access device (VAD) orders that she finds most difficult. Those orders are always more complicated than peripherally inserted central catheter (PICC) orders because PICC line orders and other VAD orders—such as Hickman, Broviac, and Groshong medication orders—do not have as many additives. Thinking of a solution with many additives reminds Courtney of total parenteral nutrition (TPN), otherwise known as hyperalimentation, which includes so many additives that they usually take up a full page of preprinted orders. Courtney gives herself a short quiz and finds that she can easily identify the common frequencies, including:

BID: twice a day	QID: four times a day
TID: three times a day	PRN: as needed or per request

Courtney has also learned that in the time since she completed school, a list of unacceptable abbreviations has been developed by the Joint Commission (JC) to identify dangerous abbreviations such as QD and QOD.

By taking some time to refresh her knowledge of medications, Courtney feels more confident that she will be able to transcribe medication orders accurately.

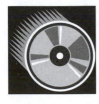

Case Scenario Questions

Based on the case scenario, define the following abbreviations.

1. TPN _____

2. VAD _____

3. BID _____

4. PO _____

5. IV _____

6. PRN _____

7. TID _____

8. PCA _____

9. PICC _____

10. IM _____

Multiple Choice Questions

1. Which of the following best describes hyperalimentation?
   a. Medications to increase the patient's blood pressure
   b. Usually given via a peripheral central catheter
   c. Usually given intramuscularly
   d. Also known as total parenteral nutrition

2. How many component parts are in a medication order?
   a. Six
   b. Five
   c. Four
   d. Three

3. Which of the following is not a component of a medication order?
   a. Name of the medication
   b. Route of the medication
   c. Color of the medication
   d. Frequency of the medication

4. The name of a medication can be which of the following?
   a. Brand name
   b. Chemical name
   c. Generic name
   d. All of the above

5. Which of the following is a drug with a two-phase system in which one liquid is dispersed throughout another liquid in the form of small droplets?
   a. Elixir
   b. Emulsion
   c. Enema
   d. Extract

6. BID is an abbreviation for which of the following?
   a. Two times a day
   b. Three times a day
   c. Four times a day
   d. Once a day

7. A PCA pump allows the patient to:
   a. Control his own blood pressure
   b. Notify the nurse that he needs pain medication
   c. Administer his own pain medication
   d. Administer his own sleep medication

8. Total parenteral nutrition feeds the patient using which of the following methods?
   a. Feeding tube
   b. Peripheral line
   c. Intravenous line
   d. Oral

9. Total parenteral nutrition is prepared in which department?
   a. Food management and nutrition services
   b. Chemistry department
   c. Nursing services
   d. Pharmacy

10. Which of the following best defines the metric system?
    a. An old European means of measurement
    b. A modern measurement system
    c. Based on the meter, kilogram, and decimal system
    d. b and c

11. A small particle or grain is known as which of the following?
    a. Film
    b. Granule
    c. Granule effervescent
    d. Inhalant

12. Which of the following is the drug form for the abbreviation "susp"?
    a. Solution
    b. Suppository
    c. Suspension
    d. Syrup

13. Which of the following describes a route that goes under the skin and into fat or connective tissue?
    a. Intradermal
    b. Transdermal
    c. Intramuscular
    d. Subcutaneous

14. Which of the following is a needle connected to a small length of tubing with a resealable cap used for intermittent infusions of small amounts?
    a. Intermittent IV
    b. Heparin lock
    c. INT line
    d. All of the above

15. Which of the following is military time for 11:30 P.M.?
    a. 1130
    b. 2130
    c. 2230
    d. 2330

16. Which of the following best describes a Schedule I controlled substance?
    a. A dangerous drug that has no recognized medical use
    b. The most dangerous drug used for medical care
    c. All locked medications
    d. The least dangerous drug

17. Which of the following is the classification of medication used to treat hypertension and fluid retention?
    a. Anticoagulant
    b. Diuretics
    c. Antianxiety
    d. Analgesic

18. Which of the following is the classification of medication used to treat nausea and vomiting?
    a. Amphetamine
    b. Antianginal
    c. Antihyperlipidemic
    d. Antiemetic

19. A 1,000 ml bag of IV fluid is to run over a 10-hour period of time. At what rate does the IV need to run?
    a. 10 ml/hour
    b. 20 ml/hr
    c. 50 ml/hr
    d. 100 ml/hr

20. The abbreviation NF is used for which of the following?
    a. No fluids
    b. Non-formulary
    c. National formulary
    d. No formula

Crossword Puzzle Medication Classifications

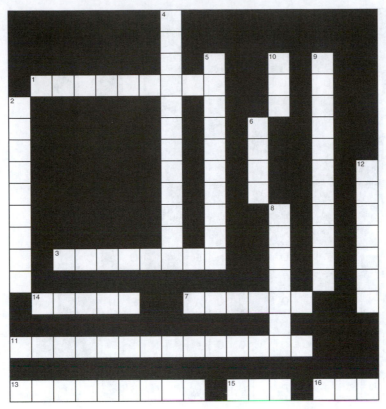

ACROSS

1. A medication that treats hypertension and fluid retention
3. Used to treat hypertension
7. Antineoplastic medications treat this disease
11. Medications used to thin blood
13. The body system that antidiabetics, corticosteroids, and thyroid medications treat
14. A five-letter abbreviation for a classification of medications used to treat inflammatory disease and pain
15. A three-letter abbreviation for the body system that the following medications treat: amphetamines, antidepressants, and analgesics
16. A three-letter abbreviation for the reference text used by physicians for medication information

DOWN

2. A classification of medications that induces sleep
4. Many medications in this group end in "-cin"
5. A common generic medication used to treat angina
6. A brand-name potassium supplement
8. A commonly used bronchodilator
9. Medications to treat nausea and vomiting
10. A three-letter abbreviation for a common medication to treat pain
12. A brand of medication used to treat arrhythmias

■ CROSSWORD PUZZLE ANSWER

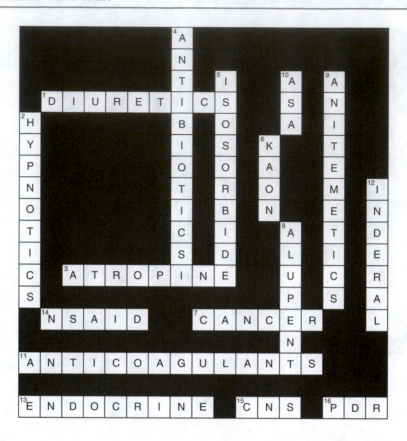

■ CASE SCENARIO ANSWERS

1. Total parenteral nutrition
2. Vascular access devices
3. Two times a day
4. By mouth
5. Intravenous
6. As necessary
7. Three times a day
8. Patient-controlled analgesia
9. Peripherally inserted central catheter
10. Intramuscular

■ MULTIPLE CHOICE ANSWERS WITH RATIONALES

1. **a.** Total parenteral nutrition is the same as hyperalimentation. (page 522)
2. **c.** Medications can be divided into four parts: name, dose, route, and frequency. (page 499)
3. **c.** Only name, dose, route, and frequency are components of medications. (page 499)
4. **d.** All medications can have a brand, chemical, and generic name. (page 500)
5. **b.** A drug with a two-phase system in which one liquid is dispersed throughout another liquid in the form of small droplets is an emulsion. (page 502)
6. **a.** "Twice a day" is abbreviated as BID. (page 511)
7. **c.** PCA is the abbreviation for "patient-controlled analgesia." (page 510)
8. **c.** Total parenteral nutrition is given via an intravenous line. (page 522)
9. **d.** Total parenteral nutrition is prepared in the pharmacy. (page 522)
10. **b.** The metric system is a modern measurement system. (page 506)
11. **b.** A small particle or grain is known as a granule. (page 502)
12. **c.** Suspension is abbreviated "susp." (page 503)
13. **d.** Subcutaneous refers to the route under the skin and into fat or connective tissue. (page 508)
14. **d.** A needle connected to a small length of tubing with a resealable cap used for intermittent infusions of small amounts can be called an intermittent IV, a heparin lock, or an INT line. (page 509)
15. **d.** 2230 is 11:30 P.M. expressed in military time. (page 513)
16. **a.** A dangerous drug that has no recognized medical use is known as a Schedule I controlled substance. (page 514)
17. **b.** Diuretics are medications used to treat hypertension and fluid retention. (page 515)
18. **d.** An antiemetic is a medication given to treat nausea and vomiting. (page 516)
19. **d.** Divide 1,000 ml by 10 hours to get 100/ml/hr. (page 522)
20. **c.** NF stands for "national formulary." (page 522)

PART E Transcribing Nursing Orders

◆ Process nursing treatment orders.

Recommended Reading

Read and review Chapters 22 and 27 of *Health Unit Coordinator: 21st Century Professional*.

Abbreviations

ECF   extended care facility

Int   intermittent

MT   empty

Sx   suction

WA   while awake

Key Terms

Bed cradle   a frame or device placed on a bed to keep bed linens from touching some part of the body

Extended care facility   a place that provides long-term nursing services for inpatients; may also be referred to as a nursing home

Foley catheter   a name for an indwelling tube inserted into the urinary bladder to continuously remove urine

CASE SCENARIO

Elmer is a certified health unit coordinator on the postsurgical wing of an extended care facility. The patients on Elmer's wing require a great deal of nursing care. A patient from a local acute care hospital has just been transferred to the wing on which Elmer works. The patient had surgery one week ago and has been transferred to the ECF for continued nursing care until the patient is ready to be discharged home.

The patient's physician has written a plan of care that includes a progressive series of nursing orders to move the patient toward independence. Elmer reads through all of the nursing orders that will direct the patient's plan of care over the next few weeks. The nursing orders are as follows:

1. Institute fall precautions
2. Check for pressure ulcers qd
3. Bed cradle for feet prn
4. Assess for signs of infections q 4h
5. Fowlers position during waking hours
6. TCDB q 2 hrs WA
7. VS qid
8. TWE prn for constipation
9. Measure fluid intake and output q 8 hrs
10. MT foley cath prn
11. Weigh qd
12. VS qid
13. Up as tol
14. Ambulate qid
15. K-pad to L. shoulder prn
16. WMC to inflamed area L arm q 4h prn
17. Sheepskin prn
18. Insert NG and connect to low int. sx as needed

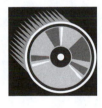

Case Scenario Questions

1. The nursing order section of the patient's Kardex is divided into the following categories:

   ◆ Activity
   ◆ Positioning
   ◆ Observation
   ◆ I/O
   ◆ Bowel elimination
   ◆ Suction
   ◆ Catheterization
   ◆ Heat/cold
   ◆ Bed

   Determine in which category of the Kardex each of the previous 18 nursing orders will be entered.

Multiple Choice Questions

1. *Pulse* is best defined as:
   a. The force of blood against the walls of the blood vessels
   b. The rate at which breathing occurs
   c. The rate at which the heart is beating
   d. The internal degree of heat of the body

2. Temperature measured in the ear is called:
   a. Tympanic
   b. Oral
   c. Axillary
   d. Rectal

3. SSE is an example of what type of order?
   a. Activity
   b. Positioning
   c. Observation
   d. Bowel elimination

4. Fall risk alert is an example of what type of order?
   a. Activity
   b. Positioning
   c. Observation
   d. Bowel elimination

5. Log roll is an example of what type of order?
   a. Activity
   b. Positioning
   c. Observation
   d. Bowel elimination

6. BRP is an example of what type of order?
   a. Activity
   b. Positioning
   c. Observation
   d. Bowel elimination

7. OOB is an example of what type of order?
   a. Activity
   b. Positioning
   c. Observation
   d. Bowel elimination

8. NG tube is an example of what type of order?
   a. Vital signs
   b. Catheterization
   c. Suction
   d. Heat/cold

9. K-pad is an example of what type of order?
   a. Vital signs
   b. Catheterization
   c. Suction
   d. Heat/cold

10. TPR is an example of what type of order?
    a. Vital signs
    b. Catheterization
    c. Suction
    d. Heat/cold

■ CASE SCENARIO ANSWERS

1. Institute fall precautions (Observation)
2. Check for pressure ulcers qd (Observation)
3. Bed cradle for feet prn (Bed)
4. Assess for signs of infections q 4h (Observation)
5. Fowler's position during waking hours (Positioning)
6. TCDB q 2 hrs WA (Activity)
7. VS qid (Observation)
8. TWE prn for constipation (Bowel elimination)
9. Measure fluid intake and output q 8 hrs (I/O)
10. MT foley cath prn (Catheterization)
11. Weigh qd (Observation)
12. VS qid (Observation)
13. Up as tol (Activity)
14. Ambulate qid (Activity)
15. K-pad to L. shoulder prn (Hot/cold)
16. WMC to inflamed area L arm q 4h prn (Hot/cold)
17. Sheepskin prn (Bed)
18. Insert NG and connect to low int. sx as needed (Catheterization)

■ MULTIPLE CHOICE ANSWERS WITH RATIONALES

1. **c.** *Pulse* is best defined as the rate at which the heart is beating. (page 481)
2. **a.** Temperature measured in the ear is called *tympanic.* (page 476)
3. **d.** Soap suds enema (SSE) is an example of a *bowel elimination* order. (page 489)
4. **c.** Fall risk alert is an example of an *observation* order. (page 486)
5. **b.** Log roll is an example of a *positioning* order. (page 485)
6. **a.** Bathroom privileges (BRP) is an example of an *activity* order. (page 483)
7. **a.** Out of bed (OOB) is an example of an *activity* order. (page 484)
8. **c.** Nasogastric (NG) tube is an example of a *suction* order. (page 490)
9. **d.** K-pad is an example of a *heat/cold* order. (page 491)
10. **a.** Temperature, pulse, and respirations (TPR) are examples of *vital signs* orders. (page 476)

CRITICAL THINKING EXERCISE

Nursing Order Equipment

Take this worksheet to a nursing unit supply area or central supply department. Identify two supplies or pieces of equipment that are used for each of the following types of orders. For example, a supply used for an observation order would be a tympanic thermometer.

1. Activity

2. Positioning

3. Observation

4. I/O

5. Bowel elimination

6. Suction

7. Catheterization

8. Heat/cold

9. Bed

For each supply or piece of equipment you identified, write an example of a nursing order in which the supply would be used. For example, a nursing order in which a tympanic thermometer would be used is "Temp QID."

PART F Surgery Orders

◆ Prepare surgical charts.

◆ Process postoperative charts.

◆ Discuss the process for preparing a surgical chart.

◆ Discuss the process for processing a postsurgical chart.

◆ Discuss post-op medication transcription.

Recommended Reading

Read and review Chapter 30 of *Health Unit Coordinator: 21st Century Professional*.

Abbreviations

ARE   advance registration and education

LIS   lab information system

OPL   outpatient laboratory

PATU   preadmission testing unit

CASE SCENARIO

Maria is a certified health unit coordinator working on the advance registration and education (ARE) unit. She is preparing surgical charts for the scheduled elective surgeries for the following day. As Maria prepares the charts, she notes that Mr. Cuez does not have the required lab reports. Maria goes to the computer and looks in the lab information system (LIS) to see if the results are available. Maria notes that there are no lab results, so she continues to check to see if they were ever ordered. Maria determines that no laboratory tests have been ordered. Maria then notifies the registered nurse, who calls Mr. Cuez and asks him to come to the outpatient laboratory (OPL) to have the labs drawn today. The policy in the OR requires that all patients have a CBC result in the chart that is not older than 30 days prior to a procedure. Mr. Cuez is scheduled to have knee replacement surgery in the morning.

At 6:30 A.M. the next day, Doreen—the certified health unit coordinator on the OPS unit—welcomes Mr. Cuez to the hospital and shows him to his room. Doreen will be double-checking Mr. Cuez's chart to make sure that all of the required reports are filed in his chart. Mr. Cuez has already signed all of the required permits, and Doreen is checking to make sure that the names and procedures are all spelled correctly and that everyone has signed in the required places. Finding everything in order, Doreen calls the holding area to let them know that Mr. Cuez has arrived and is ready to go to the OR.

At 7:30 A.M., Sally—the certified health unit coordinator in the OR—calls transport to bring Mr. Cuez to the holding area so that the OR process can begin. When Mr. Cuez arrives, Sally processes the OR paperwork and files it in the correct section of the patient chart for the health care providers in the OR.

At 9:00 A.M. Mr. Cuez is transported to the RR. Tom—the certified health unit coordinator in the RR—transcribes the RR orders and processes the paperwork. Tom enters in any charges that Mr. Cuez will have for his short stay in the RR. Tom calls the transporter to bring Mr. Cuez to the orthopedic unit.

Mr. Cuez arrives on the ortho unit at 11:00 A.M. He is brought to his room by the transporting staff. After reviewing Mr. Cruz's chart, the nurse brings it to the work-station so that the health unit coordinator can process the post-op orders.

Sarah is the certified health unit coordinator working on the ortho unit. She checks the post-op chart and sends the orders to the pharmacy so that Mr. Cuez's medication will arrive on the unit ASAP, to be given as requested by the physician.

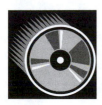

Case Scenario Questions

1. Mr. Cuez is scheduled for _____ surgery.

2. All names and procedures on the permits must be _____ correctly.

3. Medications need to arrive on the nursing unit _____ after the patient returns from surgery.

4. Testing is usually performed _____ to the patient being admitted to the health care facility if the surgery is elective.

5. Mr. Cuez's chart has been reviewed and processed by _____ health unit coordinators.

6. The _____ is Mr. Cuez's first stop after he leaves the OR.

7. Maria looks for Mr. Cuez's _____ reports in the computer system.

8. _____ is where Mr. Cuez's chart is first put together.

9. _____ orders are transcribed on the patient care unit after Mr. Cuez returns from surgery.

10. The _____ policy requires that specific lab results must be completed and on the patient chart prior to the patient being admitted to the operating room.

Multiple Choice Questions

1. Surgery that is done right away to save a patient's life is:
   a. Planned surgery
   b. Elective surgery
   c. Emergency surgery
   d. None of the above

2. A _____ _____ may be used to double-check that all required paperwork is completed prior to the patient entering the operating room.
   a. preoperative checklist
   b. patient checklist
   c. physician checklist
   d. daily checklist

3. The period after surgery is called the _____ period.
   a. perioperative
   b. preoperative
   c. postoperative
   d. interoperative

4. A physician who specializes in performing surgery is called:
   a. An oncologist
   b. A dermatologist
   c. A surgeon
   d. A doctor

5. The area where the patient waits prior to going into the operating suite is called the _____ area.
   a. waiting
   b. holding
   c. nursing
   d. none of the above

6. No _____ can be used on the surgical permit.
   a. abbreviations
   b. names
   c. ages
   d. all of the above

7. The patient may have _____ surgery scheduled through the physician's office.
   a. elective
   b. emergency
   c. irregular
   d. unplanned

8. The patient signature is required on the _____ permit unless the patient is unable to sign the permit.
   a. surgical/operative
   b. anesthesia
   c. limb disposal
   d. all of the above

9. The certified nurse who assists the anesthesiologist is:
   a. a CRNA
   b. an RNCA
   c. an LPNNA
   d. an NA

10. The patient is not able to sign the surgical permit if the patient:
    a. Has a guardian
    b. Is 24 years old
    c. Is married
    d. Has eaten lunch

CRITICAL THINKING EXERCISE

Preparing a Patient Chart for the Operating Room

1. Refer to Figures 1–1 through 1–4.

   a. Complete each permit using your name, age, and demographic
      information.

      _____

   b. Complete the pre-op checklist again, using yourself as the patient.

      _____

   If possible, repeat this exercise more than once using different people as practice
   patients undergoing different surgical procedures.

2. Using a medical dictionary, write these abbreviated procedures out as though
   you were filling out a surgical permit.

   a. TAH/BSO: _____

   b. TURP: _____

   c. Chole: _____

   d. CABG: _____

   e. GB Bx: _____

MARQUETTE GENERAL HEALTH SYSTEM
✓ CHECKLIST — ☐ SURGICAL ☐ CARDIOVASCULAR

PATIENT LABEL

UNIT CLERK RESPONSIBILITIES:
1. ____ Surgical permit on chart. Limb disposal permits (2 copies) on chart.
2. ____ Anesthesia permit signed. (Not needed for Cardiac Cath Lab) ☐ Anes. to see ☐ Parents to see Anes. ☐ Local
3. ____ Pt. in isolation—OR notified: Date:_____ Time:_____ Type of isolation:_____.
4. ____ Latex allergy—OR notified: Date:_____ Time:_____.
5. ____ Labs within 60 days. ☐ Drawn on admission.
6. ____ EKG report on chart (within 24 hrs. for Cardiac Cath Lab).
7. ____ Chest x-ray report on chart. ☐ On admission.
8. ____ History and physical on chart. ☐ MD notified ☐ To see in pre-op ☐ Other:_____.
9. ____ Old records on chart. ☐ No old records ☐ Microfilm/microfiche
10. ____ Type & screen ordered per transfusion service policy #100-028.
11. ____ Height and weight of patient entered into computer. IP.
12. ____ Height and weight of pediatric patient to pharmacy
13. ____ Pt. allergies or NKA entered into computer. IP.
14. ____ Two full pages of patient labels on inpatient chart.
15. ____ Urine or serum pregnancy test. ☐ To Lab at:_____.
16. ____ Physician Post Procedure Progress Notes placed in front of the progress notes.

CHART COMPLETED BY: _____ Date:_____ Time:_____

RN OR LPN RESPONSIBILITIES:
17. ____ Surgical permit signed. If not, please explain:_____
18. ____ Limb disposal permits signed (2 witnesses).
19. ____ ID band on non-operative side.
20. ____ Allergy band on. ____ No allergy band needed.
    Patient has latex allergies ☐ YES ☐ NO. Latex Allergy Band on _____.
21. ____ Dentures removed. (Dentures, contact lenses, glasses and hearing aid should be left on patients for Cardiac Cath Lab).
22. ____ Contact lenses or glasses removed.
23. ____ Hearing aid removed.
24. ____ Jewelry removed (O.R. notified if unable to remove). Time:_____ Person Notified:_____.
25. ____ Make-up, nail polish, hair pins and hair pieces removed.
26. ____ Head cap and gown on. (No metal snaps for Cardiac Cath Lab patients).
27. ____ Prep completed.
28. ____ Catheter in place or voided.
29. ____ Lab values within normal limits (potassium must be 3.5 or above).
30. ____ TPR and B/P taken and charted. B/P:_____ AP:_____ Temp:_____
    O_2 Sat_____ Resp._____.
31. ____ Pre-op medication given. (Administer preop sedation one hour prior to scheduled start of CABG surgery.)
32. ____ Antibiotic to be given in holding area taped to front of chart. If not why:_____.
33. ____ Chart with patient and patient ready for transport.
34. ____ Patient states hasn't had anything to eat or drink past midnight.
35. ____ Verify Surgical Site location.

Patient checked by **floor nurse**:_____ Date:_____ Time:_____

Holding Room RN verifies #32:_____ Date:_____ Time:_____

TIME OUT:
37. ____ Circulation has reviewed all information above & the surgical team agrees that they have:
    ☐ Correct Patient
    ☐ Correct Side: R_____ L_____
    ☐ Correct Site ☐ Correct Procedure ☐ Correct Position
    ☐ Correct implants/special equipment/other requirements
The permit/H&P agree with site, side & procedure to be completed.

Circulator:_____ Date:_____ Time:_____

Comments:_____

D:\IC MGH\CheckList.pmd   1/89, Rev. 3/04 MRUR-subApprove: 8/5/03   Item# 760416

Figure 1–1

MARQUETTE GENERAL HEALTH SYSTEM
Confirmation of Informed Consent

Patient Name: _____ Date of Birth: _____

The procedure, treatment or therapy is: _____

_____

_____

_____

_____

My signature on this form confirms that the general purpose, potential benefits, possible risks, complications, and inconveniences of the procedure have been explained to my satisfaction by my physician or care provider, and the alternatives have been discussed. The possible outcomes of this procedure have been explained to me, and I understand there is no guarantee that any particular result will be obtained.

I voluntarily consent to the performance of the procedure named above by:

_____ (and his/her designated

Physician/Provider Name and Title

assistants) using whatever anesthetic, treatment, medical devices, equipment, medication, or transfusion necessary. *(See back for further information).* I further authorize my physician to do what is necessary in the event that unforseen conditions arise during the course of the procedure.

I also authorize the Hospital to dispose of body parts, tissue or fluids, if removed, and/or to preserve them for diagnostic, research of teaching purposes. I agree that any photographs or video recordings, if taken, may be used for medical, scientific or educational purposes with my identify protected.

Patient, physician, or staff may add comments or explanations. Each entry should be initials and dated.

_____

_____

_____

_____

_____

_____	_____	_____	_____
Signature of Patient	Date	Signature of Witness	Date

(Signature of Parent/Guardian if patient is a minor or incompetent. Signature of Patient's Advocate as appointed under Medical Durable Power of of Attorney

(Staff Member, physician/provider's office staff, patient's family member, or other person present when patient signed)

Confirmation of Informed Consent

D:\IC MGH\ConfirmInfConsent.pm6.5P   Rev. 8/99, 1/01, 6/01, MRURsubApproved Jan. 2001

Please see other side ✍

Item # 760390

Figure 1–2a

Description of Transfusion:

Blood is introduced into one of your veins using a sterile, disposable needle. The amount of blood transfused, and whether the transfusion will be of blood, or blood components such as plasma, is a judgment your physician will make based on your particular needs.

Risks of Transfusion:

Transfusions are a common procedure of relatively low risk. Some of the risks include:
- Bruising
- Fever and Chills
- Hives or Rash
- Shortness of Breath
- Immediate or delayed transfusion reaction, including shock, heart failure,and death
- Transmission of diseases, including but not limited to infections such as hepatitis or HIV

Alternatives:

If loss of blood poses serious threats in the course of your treatment, THERE MAY BE NO EFFECTIVE ALTERNATIVE TO BLOOD TRANSFUSION. However, if you have any further questions on this matter, your physician or his/her colleagues will fully explain the alternatives to you if it has not already been done.

Figure 1–2b

MARQUETTE GENERAL HEALTH SYSTEM   PRE-ANESTHESIA EVALUATION

PERMIT FOR ANESTHESIA

I do hereby consent to any anesthesia with the exception of: _____.
I fully understand that anesthesia is not an exact science. **Major complications include, but are not limited to:** death, stroke, heart attack, paralysis, liver and kidney failure, asthma, seizures, and brain damage. **Minor complications include, but are not limited to:** Phlebitis, nerve damage, rash and/or skin damage, broken dental work and/or damaged teeth, nausea, vomiting, sore throat, head-aches, and infection. Potential adverse effects include recall of surgical events. Anesthesia at Marquette General is provided by both M.D. Anesthesiologists and Nurse Anesthetists under Anesthesiology supervision. I have received no commitment as to whom will administer my anesthetic. My signature on this form confirms that the general purpose, potential benefits, possible risks, complications, inconveniences and alternatives to care for the procedure have been explained to my satisfaction by my physician.

_____   _____   _____
Anesthesiologist/Witness   Patient or Legal Guardian   Date

NAME OF PATIENT _____

AGE _____   WEIGHT _____   HEIGHT _____

PROPOSED OPERATION _____

ALLERGIES _____

MEDICATIONS _____

ANESTHETIC HISTORY _____

_____

COULD YOU BE PREGNANT   ☐ YES   ☐ NO   ☐ NA

HISTORY OF JAUNDICE POSTSURGICAL   ☐ NO   ☐ YES _____

HISTORY OF LIVER DISEASE _____

FAMILY OR PERSONAL HISTORY OF ANESTHESIA COMPLICATIONS   ☐ NO   ☐ YES _____

H/O SMOKING   ☐ NO   ☐ YES _____   DENTAL PROBLEMS   ☐ NO   ☐ YES _____

RESPIRATORY	CARDIAC	DIABETES: ☐ NO ☐ YES
ASTHMA: ☐ NO ☐ YES	MI: ☐ NO ☐ YES	HYPERTENSION: ☐ NO ☐ YES
COPD: ☐ NO ☐ YES	ANGINA: ☐ NO ☐ YES	Kidney: _____
Auscultation _____	Auscultation _____	C.N.S. _____
HGB _____	_____	_____
OTHER: _____		

ASA Classification   1   2   3   4   5   E   **ANESTHETIC PLAN**

Patient seen and evaluated by the undersigned who agrees that patient is an appropriate candidate for proposed anesthetic.

M.D. _____   Date _____

D:\IC MGH\PermitAnesth.pm6 4/97, Rev. 10/00, 4/01, 1/02   MRURsubApprove: 01/08/02   Item # 760233

Figure 1–3

MARQUETTE GENERAL HOSPITAL
CONSENT FOR DISPOSAL OF AMPUTATED MEMBER

Date _____

Hospital No. _____

This is to certify that I, _____, consent to the

disposal of my surgically removed _____
(fill in name of member)

by the following procedure:

1) **I wish Marquette General Hospital to assume the responsibility for the disposal.**

_____
Signature of Patient

Date: _____

Witnesses:

_____

_____

2) **I wish Marquette General Hospital to release the amputated member to the**

_____ **Funeral Home.**

_____
Signature of Patient

Date: _____

Witnesses:

_____

_____

C:PROJECTS/CONSENT/AMPUTATE.DOC   4/79, Rev. 2/96

Figure 1–4

■ CASE SCENARIO ANSWERS

1. elective
2. spelled
3. ASAP
4. prior
5. five
6. RR
7. lab
8. ARE
9. post-op
10. OR

■ CRITICAL THINKING EXERCISE ANSWERS

2. a. Total abdominal hysterectomy bilateral salpingoophrectomy

   b. Transurethral resection of the prostate

   c. Cholecystectomy

   d. Coronary artery bypass graphing

   e. Gallbladder biopsy

■ MULTIPLE CHOICE ANSWERS WITH RATIONALES

1. **c.** Surgery that is done right away to save a patient's life is *emergency surgery*. (page 547)

2. **b.** A *preoperative checklist* may be used to double-check that all required paperwork is completed prior to the patient entering the operating room. (page 550)

3. **c.** The period after surgery is called the *postoperative* period. (page 557)

4. **c.** A physician who specializes in performing surgery is called *a surgeon*. (page 549)

5. **b.** The area where the patient waits prior to entering the operating suite is called the *holding* area. (page 552)

6. **a.** No *abbreviations* can be used on the surgical permit. (page 552)

7. **a.** The patient may have *elective* surgery scheduled through the physician's office. (page 549)

8. **d.** The patient signature is required on the *surgical, anesthesia,* and *limb disposal* permits unless the patient is unable to sign the permits. (page 554)

9. **a.** The certified nurse who assists the anesthesiologist is *a CRNA*. (page 557)

10. **a.** The patient is not able to sign the surgical permit if the patient *has a guardian*. (page 554)

Notification

- ◆ Notify staff of new orders.

- ◆ Notify and document consulting physicians of consult requests.

- ◆ Indicate on the order sheet that each order has been processed.

- ◆ Sign off on orders (e.g., signature, title, date, and time).

- ◆ Flag charts for cosignature.

Recommended Reading

1. Read and review Chapter 23 in *Health Unit Coordinator: 21st Century Professional*.

2. Read and review key terms at the beginning of Chapter 23 in *Health Unit Coordinator: 21st Century Professional*.

Abbreviations

DNR   do not resuscitate

Key Terms

Decentralized nursing unit   a nursing unit in which the charts are kept in an area next to the patient's room instead of at the nursing unit

Independent transcription   the health unit coordinator takes full accountability for the transcription process; the nurse does not double-check the transcribed orders

Teaching team   a team of physicians who have recently graduated and are acquiring practice in the field of medicine; a physician who is staff member of the health care facility oversees them

CASE SCENARIO

James has been a certified health unit coordinator for two years. He recently moved to a new city and has started work at a large medical center. He is still learning the names of the staff and finds he is taking more notes than he previously took when phone calls come in.

The computer system is similar to the one at his previous employer. However, James finds the process of notification of orders quite different. At his previous employer, when James entered the diets, lab tests, radiology, and other diagnostic exams—along with nursing orders and vitals signs—into the computer, they displayed on an online Kardex. At his new facility, he must remember to write in pencil *all orders* including things such as "call physician for temp greater than 102" and "vital signs every six hours."

This medical center has numerous methods of nonverbal notification that are new to James, including placing blue flags next to telephone orders that need a physician's signature and using green flags to identify new radiology orders. They use a variety of stickers on the front of charts to notify other health care facility employees that the patient has a do not resuscitate (DNR) order and/or consultation orders. They also have four different-colored stickers to identify what teaching team is following the patient.

This facility is designed with decentralized nursing units. They utilize a light system of different-colored flags outside the patient's room, used by the physician to signal that new orders have been written. There are different-colored flags for routine and stat orders, and different-colored flags to use after the orders have been transcribed. James needs to remember that when he finishes with the chart, he needs to change the flag to yellow, which notifies the nurse that the new orders have been transcribed. The flag is used in addition to James signing his name and title, and writing the date and time at the bottom of the orders, to indicate that he has completely finished the whole set of orders. James never signs off on his orders before rereading and rechecking them for accuracy. Independent transcription is also practiced at the medical center, so James must be extra careful before signing off on the orders; *independent transcription* means that the nurse does not double-check his orders for accuracy or completeness.

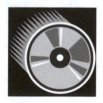

In addition to all of these methods of notification, James is keenly aware of the importance of direct verbal notification to a patient's nurse when there is a stat order written for the patient. James realizes that with time and practice, flagging and noting orders the way it is practiced at this facility will become easier.

Case Scenario Questions

1. Which of the following is an example of nonverbal communication?
   a. Turning on a lighted flag to signal that orders have been transcribed
   b. Placing a flag next to an order for a physician's signature
   c. Both a and b
   d. None of the above

2. Which of the following best defines flagging the chart for a physician's signature?
   a. Placing a consultation sticker on the front of the chart
   b. Having the nurse show the physician the order
   c. Placing a small flag next to the order
   d. Placing a phone call to the physician's office

3. Besides a health unit coordinator's name, how many other identifiers should be used to sign off on a set of orders?
   a. Two
   b. Three
   c. Four
   d. Five

4. Who is responsible for changing the flag's color after the orders have been transcribed?
   a. Nurse
   b. Physician
   c. Health unit coordinator
   d. Both a and c

5. Documentation on the Kardex must be done using what media?
   a. Black pen
   b. Red pen
   c. Pencil
   d. Both b and c

6. Which of following must the health unit coordinator do before signing and noting that the set of orders has been completed?
   a. Reread and check for accuracy
   b. Place a checkmark next to every order
   c. Place a bracket to the right of the order
   d. The nurse has read orders

7. Which of the following is not required of the health unit coordinator when signing off on orders?

    a. Time

    b. Date

    c. Title

    d. Employee number

8. Which of the following order types must always be completed immediately?

    a. Medication

    b. Admission

    c. One time

    d. Stat

9. Which of the following best defines a written note?

    a. Informal

    b. Formal

    c. Nonverbal

    d. All of the above

10. Which of the following best describes independent transcription?

    a. All transcription is done on the computer

    b. Nurses do not check and sign the orders

    c. Health unit coordinators take accountability for the transcription process

    d. Both b and c

CRITICAL THINKING EXERCISE

Notification

Take this worksheet to your facility to answer the following questions.

1. Write down all of the different tools used at your facility to notify the nursing staff of new orders.

    _____

    _____

    _____

2. Write down all of the different tools used at your facility to alert and notify other departments of patients' special needs—for example, if a patient is diabetic, blind, and a "no code."

    _____

    _____

    _____

3. Write down the steps used at your facility to notify a consulting physician.

    _____

    _____

    _____

■ CASE SCENARIO ANSWERS WITH RATIONALES

1. **d.** Utilizing any type of flagging system is a nonverbal form of communication. (page 522)

2. **c.** A flag is placed next to the order. (page 390)

3. **b.** Name, title, date, and time must be included when signing off on orders. (page 390)

4. **d.** The health unit coordinator will change the flag to notify the nurse; the nurse then changes the flag to indicate no new orders. (page 391)

5. **c.** In order to keep the Kardex current, old or completed information should be erased from it. (page 398)

6. **a.** After completing a set of orders, always go back and double-check for accuracy and thoroughness. (page 399)

7. **d.** The employee number is not necessary. (page 390)

8. **d.** Stat orders must always be processed and communicated immediately. (page 393)

9. **b.** Written communication can be formal or nonformal. (page 249)

10. **d.** Nurses do not have to check orders when independent transcription is practiced. (page 400)

■ CRITICAL THINKING EXERCISE ANSWERS

These answers provide examples of what may be used at your facility.

1. Chart flags on the outside cover of the chart, chart flags inside the chart, write the orders on a Kardex, enter the orders in the computer system, use a colored light system outside the patient's room, and verbal notification.

2. Stickers on the front cover of the chart, flags on the orders, special chart forms, and specific computer forms or communications.

3. Telephone or page the physician, use a special form in the chart, and flag the outside of the chart.

CHAPTER 3

Requests

- ◆ Request services from ancillary departments.

- ◆ Request services from support departments.

- ◆ Request supplies and equipment.

- ◆ Request patient information from external facilities.

Recommended Reading

Read and review Chapters 5, 6, 7, 9, 11, 24, 25, 26, 29, and 31 of *Health Unit Coordinator: 21st Century Professional*.

Key Terms

Ancillary   assisting in the performance of a service or the achievement of a result; used to support diagnosis and treatment of a patient's condition

Patient information from external facilities   when someone has received health care—such as services and tests—from a physician's office, clinic, hospital, or laboratory, there will be a record of care provided; the health unit coordinator will need to know how to request the records from an outside facility, including the process of obtaining the patient's permission

CASE SCENARIO

The text describes support services as services provided in the health care setting that assist the staff in providing patient care or patient assistance. Ancillary services can be defined as services that are used to support the diagnosis and treatment of a patient. Supplies and equipment are often needed to deliver care to the patient. Information about the patient's past medical treatments and tests are used by the health care team to make decisions regarding the patient's care. It takes a combination of services, supplies, and information to provide patient care. It also takes a resourceful health care team member, such as the health unit coordinator, to coordinate the many requests that result in quality patient care.

Faatimah has worked as a health unit coordinator for over five years at a university-based health system. Faatimah is a nationally certified health unit coordinator. When asked about her profession, Faatimah explains that she must know the function of every department in the system because she is the person responsible for coordinating the requests of the physicians, staff, patients, and visitors. Faatimah thinks about an average workday and guesses that she coordinates requests from at least 20 different departments. An example of some of Faatimah's responsibilities follow.

1. A patient's family member approaches Faatimah at her desk and explains that they just learned that her father must go to a nursing home.

2. A visitor asks what to do when there is a sign on the door for respiratory isolation and asks about the risks of entering the patient's room.

3. A new patient is brought to the department without any paperwork.

4. A patient has expired unexpectedly, and the patient's family is extremely distraught.

5. The nurse manager asks Faatimah to check on whether the three new employees' immunization records are up to date.

6. A physician asks for the records from a patient's previous hospitalization within the university health system.

7. A physician asks for the test results from a nuclear medicine scan that a patient had performed at a clinic outside of the university health system.

8. On her way to the laboratory, Faatimah notices that the waste can outside of the elevator is overflowing onto the floor.

9. The nurse manager asks Faatimah about the status of a new office chair that was ordered.

10. A physician informs Faatimah that a computer printer is malfunctioning. Faatimah makes several adjustments to the printer, but the printer still does not work.

11. A patient who is being discharged needs instruction on how to ambulate with a walker.

12. A nurse has a question about calculating a medication dosage.

(continued)

13. A nurse asks Faatimah to find out what type of container to use for a throat culture specimen.

14. A physician orders NG suction for a patient.

15. A patient care technician wants to know if there is a preparation for an OCG.

16. A visitor brings Faatimah a pair of eyeglasses that he found on the floor of the waiting room.

17. A nurse wants to know how much salt the patient who follows an NAS diet may have.

18. A former patient calls the department and asks Faatimah about the bill she received.

19. A patient's family member reports that a cupboard door in the patient's room is hanging off the hinges.

20. The nurse manager asks Faatimah if she can find out when the interview with a job candidate has been scheduled.

21. A nurse asks Faatimah to get information about smoking cessation classes for a patient and his wife to attend at a later date.

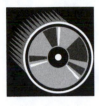

Case Scenario Questions

1. For each of the numbered situations listed in the case scenario, list where Faatimah should direct her request.

_____

_____

_____

_____

_____

_____

_____

_____

_____

_____

_____

_____

Multiple Choice Questions

1. From which department would the health unit coordinator request the development of an exercise program designed to improve mobility?

   a. Nutrition services

   b. GI lab

   c. PAS

   d. PM&R

2. From which department would the health unit coordinator request a colonoscopy?

   a. Nutrition services

   b. GI lab

   c. PAS

   d. PM&R

3. From which department would the health unit coordinator request the explanation of a restricted diet for a patient and his family?

   a. Nutrition services

   b. GI lab

   c. PAS

   d. PM&R

4. From which department would the health unit coordinator request admitting paperwork?

   a. Nutrition services

   b. GI lab

   c. PAS

   d. PM&R

5. From which department would the health unit coordinator request a reusable feeding pump?

   a. CS

   b. Environmental services

   c. HIM

   d. Purchasing

6. From which department would the health unit coordinator request the patient's medical records from a previous admission?

   a. CS

   b. Environmental services

   c. HIM

   d. Purchasing

7. From which department would the health unit coordinator request the cleaning of a patient room?

   a. CS

   b. Environmental services

   c. HIM

   d. Purchasing

8. From which department would the health unit coordinator request spiritual support services for a patient's family?

   a. HR

   b. Maintenance

   c. Pastoral care

   d. Security

9. From which department would the health unit coordinator request the storage of a patient's valuables?

   a. HR

   b. Maintenance

   c. Pastoral care

   d. Security

10. From which department would the health unit coordinator request the repair of an emergency exit light?

    a. HR

    b. Maintenance

    c. Pastoral care

    d. Security

CRITICAL THINKING EXERCISE

Ancillary and Support Departments

Take this worksheet to a nursing unit. Ask for a telephone list or directory for the health system.

1. List the names of 10 ancillary and support departments that are in the telephone directory.

   _____

   _____

   _____

   _____

   _____

   _____

   _____

   _____

   _____

   _____

2. For each of the departments listed, write an example of a request that a health unit coordinator could make from that department.

   _____

   _____

   _____

   _____

   _____

   _____

   _____

   _____

   _____

   _____

CRITICAL THINKING EXERCISE

Patient Information from External Facilities

Take this worksheet to a nursing unit. Ask for the health system's policy for obtaining patient information from external facilities. After reading the policy, answer the following questions.

1. Is a form required for the patient to give permission to obtain records?

2. If yes, obtain the form and list the name of the form.

3. Who may witness the permission or release form?

4. Are there any circumstances in which information can be obtained without a patient's permission?

5. Whose responsibility is it to contact the external facility once permission is obtained?

■ CASE SCENARIO ANSWERS

1. Social services
2. Infection control
3. Admitting or patient access services
4. Pastoral care
5. Employee health
6. Health information services or medical records
7. Check with health information services or medical records for facility policy for outside records
8. Environmental services
9. Purchasing
10. Computer services
11. Physical medicine and rehabilitation or physical therapy
12. Pharmacy
13. Clinical laboratory or bacteriology
14. Central supply
15. Diagnostic imaging or radiology
16. Security
17. Dietary or nutritional services
18. Business office or patient accounts
19. Maintenance
20. Human resources
21. Education services

■ MULTIPLE CHOICE ANSWERS WITH RATIONALES

1. **d.** Physical therapists develop exercises to improve physical mobility and work in the physical therapy department, which is a division of physical medicine and rehabilitation. (page 93)

2. **b.** A colonoscopy is a common GI department examination. (page 88)

3. **a.** Nutrition services employs registered dietitians who recommend guidelines for patients with restricted diets. (page 92)

4. **c.** The paperwork that is generated in the admitting department, also known as patient access services, accompanies the patients when they go to the nursing unit. (page 100)

5. **a.** Central supply is the department that supplies reusable patient equipment. (page 131)

6. **c.** Medical records or health information management is responsible for storing medical records and coordinating the release of information. (page 105)

7. **b.** Environmental services or housekeeping cleans and prepares the patient rooms. (page 100)

8. **c.** Pastoral care is the department that provides spiritual support. (page 101)

9. **d.** Security is the department responsible for securing valuables. (page 100)

10. **b.** Maintenance is the department responsible for maintaining and repairing the interior and exterior of the facility. (page 104)

SECTION 2

Coordination of Health Unit

CHAPTER 4

Admissions

- ◆ Label and assemble patient charts upon admission.

- ◆ Obtain patient information prior to admission.

- ◆ Assign beds to patients coming into the unit.

- ◆ Inform nursing staff of patient admission, transfer, discharge, and returning surgical patients.

- ◆ Process patient registration.

Recommended Reading

Read and review Chapter 14 of *Health Unit Coordinator: 21st Century Professional*.

Abbreviations

WIC   walk-in clinic

Key Terms

Admission board   a sheet of paper attached to a clipboard that includes a list of the names and times of admissions

Admission chart   various forms that are gathered and inserted into a binder when a patient arrives on the patient care unit

Admission packet   a collection of information that contains all of the forms required to admit a patient to the patient care unit

Bed control   a daily meeting that a unit representative attends along with the other units and the admitting department representative to discuss the planned admissions and discharges for that day and the next

Charge nurse   the nurse who receives reports on all patients for a given unit and assists with nursing decisions for a given day when the nurse manager is unavailable

Planned admission   a patient whose date and time of arrival have been arranged prior to arrival; also called a *scheduled admission*

CASE SCENARIO

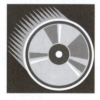

The surgical unit on 4 West is a busy unit during the week. Today is Tuesday, and Maria, a health unit coordinator, is arriving at 6:30 A.M. to start her shift. She knows that yesterday, at bed control, there were four planned admissions scheduled for today. When Maria arrives at the workstation to start her shift, she checks the admission board to see who the admissions are for today. There are now five admissions listed. The first admission is scheduled to arrive at 6:45 A.M. Maria pulls five chart holders (or binders) and five admission packets. The first admission arrives and Maria asks the assigned nurse to take the patient to his room. Two admissions are scheduled to arrive at 7:00 A.M. and both arrive at the workstation at the same time. Maria takes one admission to her room and asks the assigned nurse to take the other admission to his room. When Maria returns to the workstation, she processes the chart for the patient who will be going to the OR first. Maria checks the OR schedules to make sure that she is completing the admission chart for the correct patient. The admitting department calls Maria to notify her that a patient in the walk-in clinic (WIC) needs to be admitted to her unit ASAP. Maria gives the information regarding the patient to the charge nurse, who will decide what room to assign the patient. The patient will be placed in a room that was to be used for one of the scheduled admissions expected to arrive at 1:00 P.M. Maria hopes that the family of the patient in room 404 arrives soon and that housekeeping will be able to clean the room before the 1:00 P.M. admission arrives, so that the new patient can be placed promptly. The day has only just begun, and the admission board has already been changed twice. Looks like it will be a busy day on the surgical unit.

Case Scenario Questions

Based on the case scenario, determine whether the following statements are true or false.

1. Patients can be admitted from WIC to the surgical unit.

2. There are four planned admissions for today.

3. Maria processes the admission that is going to surgery first when two admissions arrive at the same time.

4. Only planned admissions are admitted to the surgical unit.

5. Maria decides which room the patient from WIC will use.

6. Maria gets ready for the patient admissions by pulling the admission packets prior to the patients arriving on the unit.

7. Only the patient's nurse can take patients to their assigned rooms.

8. The surgical unit is having a busy day.

9. Maria can check the OR schedule for the times that patients are scheduled to go to the OR.

10. Maria can attend bed control.

Multiple Choice Questions

1. _____ is a component of the admission process.
   a. Registration
   b. Communication
   c. Technology
   d. Priority

2. Once a patient is registered in the health care system, the registration is considered _____.
   a. completed
   b. processed
   c. single
   d. new

3. _____ admissions are most often transported by EMS personnel.
   a. Direct
   b. Scheduled
   c. Regular
   d. Surgical

4. The most common patient admission types are inpatient, _____, short-stay patients, and same-day patients.
   a. prepatients
   b. outpatients
   c. x-patients
   d. postpatients

5. A(n) _____ admission is a planned admission.
   a. scheduled
   b. direct
   c. emergency
   d. none of the above

6. The signed patient _____ form gives the health care system permission to treat the patient and bill the patient's insurance company.
   a. signature
   b. permission
   c. consent
   d. health

7. A(n) _____ admission is admission of a patient that has not been preplanned by the patient.
   a. unscheduled
   b. elective
   c. regular
   d. scheduled

8. The patient _____ _____ is a form that contains information about the patient and is completed by the nursing staff.
   a. medical record
   b. data base
   c. advance directive
   d. none of the above

9. _____ is the abbreviation for "against medical advice."
   a. MA
   b. AMA
   c. AGMA
   d. AMAD

10. A copy of the advance directive is kept in the patient's _____.
    a. room
    b. chart
    c. closet
    d. drawer

CRITICAL THINKING EXERCISE

Patient Admissions

1. Visit the Web sites of the health care facilities in your community.

   a. Find the number of admissions that each facility has in a year.

   b. Search for the online patient registration form for each facility. Print the form and review it.

   c. List three things that the patient can complete on the form prior to admission.

2. Call the admitting department of one of your local health care facilities and ask them to send you the materials that they send to all scheduled admissions. Review the information. Is there information about:

   a. Visiting hours?

   b. Advance directives?

   c. Home medications?

■ CASE SCENARIO ANSWERS

1. True
2. True
3. True
4. False
5. False
6. True
7. False
8. True
9. True
10. True

■ MULTIPLE CHOICE ANSWERS WITH RATIONALES

1. **a.** *Registration* is a component of the admission process. (page 212)

2. **b.** A registration is considered *processed* once the patient is registered into the health care registration system. (page 214)

3. **a.** *Direct* admissions are most often transported by emergency medical service (EMS) employees. (page 218)

4. **b.** The common patient types include inpatients, *outpatients,* same-day patients, and short-stay patients. (page 229)

5. **a.** A *scheduled* admission is a planned admission. (page 217)

6. **c.** The signed patient *consent* form gives the health care system permission to treat the patient and bill the patient's insurance company. (page 214)

7. **a.** An *unscheduled* admission is admission of a patient who did not plan to be admitted to the health care facility. (page 217)

8. **b.** The patient *data base* is a form completed by the nursing staff that contains information about the patient. (page 222)

9. **b.** *AMA* is the abbreviation for "against medical advice." (page 211)

10. **b.** A copy of the patient's advance directive is kept in the patient's *chart.* (page 227)

CHAPTER 5

Patient Results Processing

- ◆ Receive diagnostic test results.

- ◆ Notify physicians of diagnostic test results.

- ◆ Report diagnostic test results to nursing staff.

Recommended Reading

1. Read and review Chapters 15, 16, and 24 of *Health Unit Coordinator: 21st Century Professional*.

2. Read and review the key terms at the beginning of Chapter 23 in *Health Unit Coordinator: 21st Century Professional*.

CASE SCENARIO

Iris is a certified health unit coordinator in a busy emergency department. In addition to ordering tests in an efficient manner, processing the test results promptly and accurately is an important task for Iris. Often the results are retrievable from the medical center's computer system. Iris is familiar with the different applications and screens she can use to find lab results quickly. However, when the computer system crashes, Iris has the more challenging task of taking results over the telephone. This is the same challenge that faces health unit coordinators who work the nursing units of the medical center. When the diagnostic departments call with results, Iris must give her full attention, concentrating *only* on the call for a few minutes. She must not be preoccupied with anything else while she is on the phone. She will write down the name of the patient, the test results as spoken by the caller, and the caller's name, and repeat back the results for verification. The last two steps—documenting the caller's name and repeating back the results—are recommendations from the Joint Commission (JC). As soon as Iris receives the results, she must find either the patient's nurse or the physician and promptly deliver the results to them. Handing off, or communicating, the results must be done so only the health care worker will hear the conversation.

In a busy area like the emergency room, it is helpful for Iris to have an understanding of some of the more critical tests and their normal ranges (for adults), such as:

- Potassium   3.5–5.3
- Sodium   135–145
- Chloride   98–106
- Prothrombin time (PT)   11.0–13.0 sec
- Partial thromboplastin time (PTT)   21–35 sec
- Hemoglobin
    - Women   12.0–16.0
    - Men   14.0–17.4
- Hematocrit
    - Women   36%–48%
    - Men   42%–52%

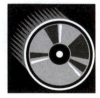

If results are sent to the unit printer while the patient is still in the emergency room, it is crucial that Iris place the results in the correct patient's chart and in the correct area of the chart; in other words, she must ensure that PTs and PTTs get filed with lab reports, that a KUB gets filed with radiology or imaging reports, and so forth.

Case Scenario Questions: True/False

1. Iris needs to avoid distractions when she is on the telephone taking results.

2. Lab results can be printed on the nursing unit and called to the unit by lab personnel.

3. Iris knows the normal ranges for common lab tests.

4. Since Iris works in the emergency room, she does not need to file test results.

5. Since Iris works in the emergency room, it is okay for her to *just verbally* notify the nurse of test results as they are called in.

6. A normal PTT level is 21–35 sec.

7. A normal H & H is different for men and women.

8. KUB results should be filed in the front of the chart while the patient is in the emergency room.

9. JC is the abbreviation for Joint Commission.

10. Radiology and imaging are the same department.

Multiple Choice Questions

1. Who can take diagnostic results over the telephone?

   a. Physicians

   b. Nurses

   c. Health unit coordinators

   d. Consult your employer's policy

2. Which of the following is the best way to receive diagnostic test results over the telephone?

   a. Write down the test results and give them to the patient's nurse.

   b. Write down the test results, along with the caller's name, and give them to the patient's nurse.

   c. Write down the name of the patient, the test results, and the caller's name, and repeat back the results for verification.

   d. Both a and b

3. The JC makes which of the following for health care facilities?

   a. Laws

   b. Recommendations

   c. Rules

   d. Policies

4. Which of the following should be done while taking lab results over the telephone?

   a. Flag down the patient's nurse.

   b. Flag down the physician.

   c. Watch for visitors.

   d. Do not be preoccupied with anything.

5. Which of the following should be done if results are called in that are not within the normal limits?

   a. Quickly but quietly relay the message to the patient's nurse or physician.

   b. Using the intercom, dial into the patient's room and relay the results.

   c. Give the results to any available nurse in the nurse's station.

   d. Send the results via the call system.

6. The normal range for a sodium level is which of the following?

   a. 100–125

   b. 125–134

   c. 135–145

   d. 145–165

7. The normal range for a chloride level is which of the following?

   a. 98–106

   b. 106–125

   c. 126–150

   d. 151–160

8. The normal range for potassium is which of the following?

   a. 2.0–3.5

   b. 3.5–5.0

   c. 3.0–6.0

   d. 4.0–7.0

9. Nonverbal communication should only be used in which of the following situations?

   a. Outside of a hospital setting

   b. Never in an emergency room

   c. Whenever you want

   d. When it is easier and faster than verbal communication

10. The normal range for a prothrombin time is which of the following?

    a. 9.00–11.0 sec

    b. 11.0–13.0 sec

    c. 13.0–15.0 sec

    d. 15.0–17.0 sec

■ CASE SCENARIO ANSWERS

1. True
2. True
3. True
4. False
5. False
6. True
7. True
8. False
9. True
10. True

■ MULTIPLE CHOICE ANSWERS WITH RATIONALES

1. **d.** Consult your facility procedures regarding test results procedures. (page 388)
2. **c.** Write down the test results and the caller's name, and repeat back the results for verification. (page 388)
3. **b.** The JC makes *recommendations* for health care facilities to follow. (page 388)
4. **d.** When taking results over the phone, never be preoccupied with anything else. (page 259)
5. **a.** Quickly but quietly relay the message to the patient's nurse or physician. (page 259)
6. **c.** The normal range for a sodium level is *135–145.* (*Manual of Laboratory and Diagnostic Tests*)
7. **a.** The normal range for a chloride level is *98–106.* (*Manual of Laboratory and Diagnostic Tests*)
8. **b.** The normal range for a potassium level is *3.5–5.0.* (*Manual of Laboratory and Diagnostic Tests*)
9. **d.** Nonverbal communication can be used when it is easier and faster than verbal communication. (page 253)
10. **b.** The normal range for a prothrombin time is *11.0–13.0.* (*Manual of Laboratory and Diagnostic Tests*)

CHAPTER 6

Discharges/Transfers

- ◆ Assemble necessary forms and perform clerical tasks for patients being transferred to an external facility.

- ◆ Prepare patient charts and perform clerical tasks for discharge or transfer to other units within the health facility.

- ◆ Notify appropriate departments and individuals when patients are discharged (e.g., home, expired, AMA, transferred, etc.).

- ◆ Disassemble patient charts, put in appropriate order, and send to medical records office upon expiration or discharge.

- ◆ Schedule follow-up appointments.

- ◆ Schedule appointments for diagnostic work at other facilities.

- ◆ Follow organ procurement procedures.

- ◆ Schedule ground transportation for patients.

Recommended Reading

Read and review Chapter 14 of *Health Unit Coordinator: 21st Century Professional*.

Abbreviations

BMP   basic metabolic panel

Appt   appointment

Chem7   chemistry 7

F/U   follow-up

H/A   headache

Meds   medications

PLU   patient left unit

Rx   prescription

Key Terms

Basic Metabolic Panel   seven chemistry tests including CO_2, Cl, Na, K, Ca, BUN, and glucose that are ordered as one panel of tests

CASE SCENARIO

Rosa is a newly hired, certified health unit coordinator working on the medical unit with Sarah, a 10-year veteran certified health unit coordinator. Rosa has Mr. Brown's chart, which contains the following orders written by Dr. Hungee:

1. Discharge to home
2. Appt in office in 2 weeks for F/U with BMP
3. Discharge meds:

   Lanoxin 0.25 mg po daily

   ASA 81 mg po daily

   Tylenol 650 mg Q 4 hrs prn H/A

Rosa completes the order, including writing the discharge medications on the patient discharge summary. Sarah reviews Rosa's transcribed orders, checking for the following items prior to cosigning Rosa's orders:

1. She checks to make sure that the planned discharge is written on the patient census and that the charge nurse is aware that the patient is going home.
2. She checks for the doctor's appointment slip and that it is completed correctly. She also checks that the date and time of the physician appointment are written on the discharge summary.
3. She checks that the laboratory test request for a BMP is written on the discharge summary and that the outpatient laboratory request for the BMP is labeled with the patient's name and correctly filled out. She makes sure it is attached to the discharge summary.
4. She checks to make sure that there is an Rx written for each medication ordered that requires an Rx, and that this is attached to the discharge summary.
5. She checks to make sure that all of the discharge meds are written on the discharge summary in layperson language. Example: *po* is written as "orally," and *daily* is written as "once a day."

Sarah explains to Rosa that when Mr. Brown's family arrives to take him home and the nurse has completed reviewing the discharge instructions with Mr. Brown, she will need to PLU the patient in the computer system.

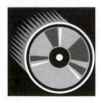

After the patient has been discharged, Rosa will take the patient chart apart and put all of the papers in the correct order for the HIM department.

Case Scenario Questions

1. After the patient is discharged, the _____ department requires that the papers be put in the correct order.

2. Sarah is a _____ unit coordinator who cosigns the new health unit coordinator's transcription.

3. The F/U _____ is written on the discharge summary.

4. Discharge information must be written in _____ language.

5. _____ is a discharge medication that can be used for H/A by Mr. Brown.

6. Mr. Brown has a return appointment to see Dr. _____.

7. All patients are _____ when they are discharged and leave the nursing unit.

8. Each medication ordered may need to have a written _____.

9. In layperson language, *po* would be written as _____.

10. Rosa and Sarah are working on the _____ unit.

Multiple Choice Questions

1. Both the patient and the care provider who review the discharge summary with the patient must _____ the summary.
   a. sign
   b. review
   c. both a and b
   d. none of the above

2. Following some deaths, the _____ requires an autopsy.
   a. family
   b. nurse
   c. law
   d. physician

3. All patients are provided with discharge _____.
   a. instructions
   b. drugs
   c. supplies
   d. foods

4. Patients can be discharged to another facility, such as a(n):
   a. Extended care facility
   b. Jail
   c. Halfway house
   d. All of the above

5. The health unit coordinator will _____ the patient's chart when the patient is discharged.
   a. file
   b. assemble
   c. disassemble
   d. review

6. Some patients are discharged to home but still require _____ care.
   a. nursing
   b. extended
   c. daily
   d. health

7. When the patient chart arrives in the HIM department, the _____ process begins.
   a. admission
   b. discharge
   c. filing
   d. coding

8. The surrounding area of a health care facility is defined by _____.
   a. EMTALA
   b. TLAMA
   c. ETTALMA
   d. none of the above

9. It is important that the discharge information be written in _____ that the patient can read and understand.
   a. code
   b. a language
   c. English
   d. medical jargon

10. A(n) _____ is the process of moving a patient from one location to another location.
    a. admission
    b. transfer
    c. slide
    d. none of the above

CRITICAL THINKING EXERCISE

Health Care Facilities and Services

1. Call your local home health services and ask the following questions:

   a. What types of services do you provide?

   b. What is your service area?

   c. What is the fee structure?

   Ask for additional information to be mailed to your home.

   _____

   _____

   _____

2. Look either on the Web or in the yellow pages to see how many extended care facilities and nursing homes are in your area. If possible, call one of the facilities and ask to talk with an admission nurse or social worker. Ask the following questions:

   a. Where do your patients come from: hospitals, homes, or other facilities?

   b. What services do you provide (e.g., PT, OT, etc.)?

   Ask for additional information to be mailed to your home.

   _____

   _____

   _____

   Make a comparison chart of the information you gathered and write your conclusions. For example, describe the types of services that are provided by all of the facilities, the different price ranges, and so forth.

■ CASE SCENARIO ANSWERS

1. HIM
2. veteran
3. appointment
4. layperson
5. Tylenol
6. Hungee
7. PLU
8. Rx (prescription)
9. orally
10. medical

■ MULTIPLE CHOICE ANSWERS AND RATIONALE

1. **a.** The patient and the care provider both review and sign the discharge summary. (page 236)
2. **c.** In some death cases, the law requires an autopsy. (page 242)
3. **a.** All patients discharged from the health care facility are provided with discharge instructions. (page 236)
4. **d.** Patients can be discharged to other facilities that include assisted-living facilities, jails, prisons, and halfway houses. (page 239)
5. **c.** After the patient is discharged from the patient care unit, the health unit coordinator disassembles the patient chart. (page 239)
6. **a.** Some patients are discharged to home and still require nursing care. (page 239)
7. **d.** When the discharged chart arrives in the HIM department (medical records), the coding process begins. (page 239)
8. **a.** The Emergency Medical Treatment and Active Labor Act (EMTALA) defines the surrounding area of a health care facility. (page 239)
9. **b.** It is important that the discharge instructions be written in a language that the patient can read and understand. (page 236)
10. **b.** The process of moving a patient from one location to another is called a transfer. (page 230)

CHAPTER 7

Unit Responsibilities: Clerical

- ◆ Maintain a supply of chart forms.

- ◆ Maintain stock of patient care supplies and equipment.

- ◆ Maintain stock of clerical and desk supplies.

- ◆ Maintain patient charts by thinning and adding forms as needed.

- ◆ File forms and reports.

- ◆ Maintain unit bulletin board.

- ◆ Maintain policy and procedures manuals.

- ◆ Monitor patients' off-unit locations.

- ◆ Arrange for maintenance and repair of equipment.

Recommended Reading

Read and review Chapters 5, 9, 13, 16, and 31 of *Health Unit Coordinator: 21st Century Professional.*

Key Terms

Indirect patient care   nonclinical duties performed without having direct physical contact with the patient

CASE SCENARIO

Donnalyn is a certified health unit coordinator on the neurological unit. Because of her experience and patience, she is often asked to train new staff. For the past few weeks, Donnalyn has been working with a new employee, Patrick. Patrick is a nursing student who is working as a health unit coordinator while he is attending school. Donnalyn has observed that Patrick transcribes orders accurately, but he hasn't yet demonstrated a full understanding of the importance of his other job duties.

As a health unit coordinator, Donnalyn performs the clerical responsibilities on the unit in addition to transcribing physician orders. Donnalyn knows there are certain tasks that must be performed to maintain a well-functioning unit. These tasks are often referred to as *clerical tasks* or *indirect patient care*. For example, it is the health unit coordinator's responsibility to update the policy and procedures manuals. On a regular basis, the unit coordinator adds the updated policies and removes the outdated policies from the manuals. It is also the health unit coordinator's responsibility to file reports in the patients' medical records. Reports from laboratory and diagnostic imaging departments may be sent to the unit by facsimile, computer, or pneumatic tube. The health unit coordinator files these reports in the patients' charts in a timely manner. Other clerical or indirect patient care tasks include maintaining a supply of chart forms, stock of patient care supplies and equipment, stock of clerical and desk supplies, patient charts (by thinning and adding forms as needed), the unit bulletin board, and policy and procedures manuals. The health unit coordinator is also responsible for monitoring patients' off-unit locations and arranging for the maintenance and repair of equipment.

Donnalyn believes that Patrick must understand the importance of the clerical tasks to be a successful health unit coordinator. Donnalyn surveys the workstation and notices that many clerical tasks haven't been completed. She writes a list of the unfinished tasks, as follows:

1. There are no neurological vital signs chart forms in the cupboard.
2. Two patient charts are missing from the chart rack and cannot be found at the workstation.
3. An IV pole with a broken wheel is in the utility room.
4. An e-mail announcement was sent to the unit that the policy for hand-washing techniques had been updated. A copy of the revised policy is still attached to the e-mail.
5. A respiratory therapist reported that there were no extra progress notes in his patients' charts.
6. The fax machine is out of paper.
7. An overhead light in the hallway has burned out.
8. One of the younger patients takes his po medications with sherbet, but the unit's patient nourishment freezer is empty.

(continued)

9. A stack of radiology reports that were received during the previous shift is on the countertop of the workstation.

10. One of the patient's charts is so full that it no longer fits in the chart rack and the chart binder rings barely close.

11. The mandatory safety class schedule posted on the bulletin board is two months old.

12. A nurse complains that there are no sterile specimen cups in the storage cupboard for the stat urine culture she is to obtain.

Donnalyn shows the list of unfinished tasks to Patrick. Patrick responds that it is his job to transcribe orders and that these other tasks are unimportant. Donnalyn is unsure of what to do next.

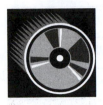

Case Scenario Questions

1. For each of the previous tasks, write how you would explain to Patrick that each of the clerical tasks affects patient care and safety.

_____

_____

_____

_____

_____

_____

_____

_____

_____

_____

_____

_____

_____

_____

_____

2. For each of the previous tasks, write the action Patrick should take to complete it.

_____

_____

_____

_____

_____

_____

_____

_____

_____

_____

_____

_____

_____

_____

_____

Multiple Choice Questions

1. Which of the following is the term given to items that are used by the health unit coordinator to carry out the requirements of the job?
   a. Manual charges
   b. Reusable equipment
   c. Services
   d. Supplies

2. Which of the following can lead to a delay in patient care?
   a. Faulty equipment
   b. Missing supplies
   c. Both a and b
   d. None of the above

3. What is another name for the central supply department?
   a. Print shop
   b. Purchasing
   c. Sterile processing and distribution
   d. Unit utility room

4. What term describes the practice of pulling out certain forms from a patient's chart because the record has become too large to handle?
   a. Dividing
   b. Separating
   c. Stuffing
   d. Thinning

5. Which of the following is an air-operated system in which small items can be transported via a cylindrical carrier?
   a. Pneumatic tube system
   b. Automatic dispenser system
   c. Air canister system
   d. Air filtration system

6. Supplies may be ordered by:
   a. Computer entry
   b. Paper or written requisition
   c. Both a and b
   d. None of the above

7. Which of the following practices, when done in advance, helps the staff by making sure that they have the necessary forms at hand in the patient chart?
   a. Thinning
   b. Stuffing
   c. Augmenting
   d. Padding

8. With regard to the process of ordering supplies, the health unit coordinator should have:
   a. A procedure for how to order
   b. A system in place to alert that a supply is low
   c. A determined time frame in which to order
   d. All of the above

9. Which of the following is the form used to request supplies from an outside vendor?
   a. PO
   b. SPD
   c. CS
   d. CPD

10. Which of the following is a reusable piece of equipment that is rented for a specific amount of time?
    a. IV needle and tubing
    b. IV pump
    c. IV solution
    d. IV tape

CRITICAL THINKING EXERCISE

Clerical Responsibilities

1. List two methods by which supplies may be delivered to the workstation.

   _____

   _____

2. List three pieces of information that should be recorded in the sign in/out board.

   _____

   _____

3. Name the department within the facility that is responsible for the equipment rented or purchased by the patient.

   _____

   _____

4. List two chart forms that may be added to the patient's chart in advance of use.

   _____

   _____

5. List three methods used to communicate requests to the maintenance department.

   _____

   _____

6. List three types of clerical supplies.

   _____

   _____

7. List three types of information that may be posted on the unit bulletin board.

   _____

   _____

CRITICAL THINKING EXERCISE

Supplies

1. Arrange for a tour of the following departments: purchasing, central supply, print shop, and linen. Take this worksheet with you on your tours. For each department that you tour, list examples of supplies and the methods used to request the supplies.

   _____

   _____

   _____

   _____

2. Take this worksheet to a nursing unit and arrange for a tour of the storage areas. Make a list of where each of the following types of supplies, equipment, or forms is stored.

   a. Chart forms _____

   b. Clerical supplies _____

   c. One-time-use patient supplies _____

   d. Reusable patient supplies _____

   e. Nutrition supplies _____

   f. Broken equipment _____

   g. Used or dirty reusable equipment _____

   h. Reports to be filed _____

   i. Policy and procedures manual _____

   j. Bulletin board _____

   k. Sign in/out board _____

3. For the following types of supplies, list the method that the health unit coordinator utilizes to keep track of when the supply is running low, how often the supplies are ordered, and the method used to order them.

   a. Chart forms _____

   b. Clerical supplies _____

   c. One-time-use patient supplies _____

   d. Reusable patient supplies _____

   e. Nutrition supplies _____

■ CASE SCENARIO SUGGESTED ANSWERS

1. Without the correct form in the chart, the documentation of observations may be compromised. Patrick should order a supply of forms from the print shop.

2. The health unit coordinator must know the location of the patients' charts at all times to protect confidentiality. Patrick should locate the charts and update the sign in/out board if necessary.

3. Faulty equipment can delay patient care. Patrick should request repair from the maintenance department.

4. Patients and staff may be in danger without access to current policies. Patrick should place the updated policy in the correct manual, remove the outdated policy, and post a copy of the new policy on the bulletin board. All of this should be done in accordance with the facility's policy.

5. Without the correct forms in the charts, the documentation of observations may be compromised. Patrick should make time to stuff the patients' charts.

6. Missing supplies can delay patient care. Patrick should replenish the paper supply in the fax machine.

7. Faulty equipment can delay patient care. Patrick should request repair from the maintenance department.

8. Missing supplies can delay patient care. Patrick should review the nutrition inventory and order the necessary food items.

9. Without current reports available, patient care may be compromised or delayed. Patrick should find time to file the reports in the patients' charts.

10. An overstuffed chart may result in lost forms. Patrick should thin the chart according to policy.

11. Patients and staff may be in danger without access to current schedules for mandatory classes. Patrick should remove the outdated information from the bulletin board and look to see if updated information is available to post. All of this should be done in accordance with the facility's policy.

12. Missing supplies can delay patient care. Patrick should review the patient supply inventory and order the necessary supplies.

■ MULTIPLE CHOICE ANSWERS WITH RATIONALES

1. **d.** Supplies is the term given to items that are used by the health unit coordinator to carry out the requirements of the job. (page 126)

2. **c.** Both faulty equipment and missing supplies can lead to a delay in patient care. (page 72)

3. **c.** Sterile processing and distribution is another name for the central supply department. (page 126)

4. **d.** Thinning is the term given to the practice of pulling our certain forms from a patient's charge because the record has become too large to handle. (page 207)

5. **a.** An air-operated system in which small items can be transported in a cylindrical carrier is called a pneumatic tube system. (page 274)

6. **c.** Supplies may be ordered by computer or written paper requisition. (page 127)

7. **b.** Stuffing is the practice done ahead of time to help the caregivers by making sure they have the necessary forms at hand. (page 100)

8. **d.** With regard to the process of ordering supplies, the health unit coordinator should have a procedure for how to order, a system in place to alert that a supply is low, and a determined time frame in which to order. (page 127)

9. **a.** A purchase order (PO) is the name of the form that is used to request supplies from an outside vendor. (page 128)

10. **b.** An IV pump is a reusable piece of equipment that is rented for a specific amount of time. (page 131)

■ CRITICAL THINKING EXERCISE ANSWERS

1. Pneumatic tube and dumbwaiter (page 74)

2. Time of departure, destination, and name of transporter (page 76)

3. Central supply or sterile processing and distribution (page 125)

4. Physician's order form and progress notes (page 193)

5. Computer program, telephone call, and written request (page 577)

6. Writing instruments, paper chart forms, paper clips, tape, or computer supplies (page 127)

7. Staff schedules, policy updates, and health system changes and updates (page 278)

CHAPTER 8

Reports and Record Keeping

- ◆ Report unit activities to incoming shift.

- ◆ Maintain patient census logs.

- ◆ Record patient acuity.

- ◆ Record unit/department statistics.

- ◆ Graph and chart information onto appropriate forms.

- ◆ Maintain patient census boards and communication boards.

- ◆ Maintain on-call schedules.

- ◆ Maintain patient assignment board.

- ◆ Perform quality assurance on charts (i.e., verify that chart forms are filed and labeled correctly, all orders have been transcribed, allergies are noted in appropriate places, all incident reports are prepared, etc.).

- ◆ Reconcile patient charges/credits.

- ◆ Retrieve test results.

- ◆ Recopy medication administration records.

- ◆ Recopy Kardex/patient treatment plan.

- ◆ Inventory unit equipment.

Recommended Reading

Read and review Chapters 5, 9, and 23 of *Health Unit Coordinator: 21st Century Professional.*

CASE SCENARIO

Sid works the second shift on a medical surgical nursing unit that has a maximum capacity of 40 patients. Some days there may be 10 discharges, 6 surgical admissions, and numerous tests and procedures scheduled for the balance of the patients. Sid needs to know where the patients are at all times, which patients have been discharged or admitted, and which tests have or have not been completed. If tests have not been completed, Sid usually needs to reschedule them. If the patient is to have a paracentesis, Sid needs to pull a consent form, make sure the paracentesis tray is on the unit, and communicate the order to the patient's nurse. Once the paracentesis is completed, Sid will need to send the fluid down to lab with the appropriate labels, enter the charges for the paracentesis tray, and call central service to replace the paracentesis tray.

When the unit gets this busy, there is only one way Sid can manage it: by *staying organized*. From the very beginning of her orientation, organizational skills were stressed to Sid. She uses numerous tools to ensure organization, including the following.

At the beginning of her shift, Sid receives the report from the first shift. She writes notes regarding expected activities for the patients on the *census list* next to the appropriate patient name and always adds names to the *census board* as soon as a patient is admitted. Sid makes sure that the *patient activity board* is always nearby, in case someone comes to the desk looking for a patient. The patient activity board can also be used to see if a patient has been taken to a department for a particular test during the day shift.

As she transcribes orders, Sid knows that it is important for her to update (*in pencil*, so she can erase outdated orders) the patient Kardex so that the nurses are aware of new patient orders—not just exams, but also diets, treatments and activity and observation orders, which can change quickly.

Part of the second shift health unit coordinator's routine responsibilities are to graph patient's vital signs, ensure that patient acuities are entered into the computer, make sure that the *patient assignment board* is current, enter charges and recopy Kardexes and medication administration records (MARs), check the inventory of unit equipment, and order additional equipment as necessary.

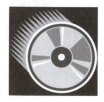

On weekend evenings, Sid is expected to record unit statistics, update the *on-call schedules,* and perform quality assurance on charts to verify that all chart forms are labeled correctly, all orders have been transcribed, and allergies are noted in the appropriate places.

Case Scenario Questions: True/False

1. Since Sid works full time on the second shift, she does not need to take notes during the shift report.

2. Completing a patient's Kardex using red ink is encouraged, since the nurse will note the red ink more easily.

3. Treatment and observation orders should only be entered on the Kardex by the nurse.

4. Health unit coordinators should do quality assurance audits on charts.

5. Health unit coordinators need to know all the different places on a chart that should be flagged for allergies.

6. It is important for health unit coordinators to update the Kardex so they know where the patient is at all times.

7. Diets and medications need not be written on a Kardex.

8. All changes in a patient's activity status must be written on a Kardex.

9. Only nurses can record acuities for patients.

10. Only nurses can graph a patient's vital signs and I & O in the patient's medical record.

Multiple Choice Questions

1. Which answer best defines the type of charging systems that can be found in health care facilities?
   a. Computerized
   b. Manual
   c. Both computerized and manual
   d. All of the above

2. What type of shift report do health unit coordinators receive?
   a. Clinical
   b. Nonclinical
   c. Both a and b
   d. None of the above

3. Which of the following is a charge for equipment used on a daily basis for a patient?
   a. Service charge
   b. Equipment charge
   c. Purchase order
   d. Daily charge

4. Which of the following is a charge generated to the patient bill for goods, services, or equipment?
   a. Service charge
   b. Patient charge
   c. Purchase charge
   d. Equipment charge

5. Which of the following is used to place orders from an outside vendor?
   a. Purchase order
   b. Patient requester
   c. Phone order
   d. Vendor order

6. Patient acuity reflects which of the following?
   a. The severity of the patient's condition and the level of care needed for the patient
   b. The severity of the patient's condition and the number of staff needed to care for the patient
   c. The severity of the patient's condition
   d. The level of care needed for the patient

7. Which member of the staff is responsible for the upkeep of the unit census?
   a. Nurse manager
   b. Health unit coordinator
   c. Charge nurse
   d. Admitting department

8. Which type of visitor request can the health unit coordinator handle?
   a. Concern about the patient's pain level
   b. Concern about the temperature of the patient's room being too cold
   c. Condition of the patient
   d. Hospital policy on visitor hours

9. Which of the following is the order classification for a treatment order?
   a. Therapy
   b. Nursing care
   c. Medication
   d. Miscellaneous

10. Which of the following is the order classification for a neurophysiology order?
    a. Nursing care
    b. Diagnostic procedure
    c. Therapy
    d. Miscellaneous

■ CASE SCENARIO ANSWERS

1. False
2. False
3. False
4. True
5. True
6. False
7. False
8. True
9. False
10. False

■ MULTIPLE CHOICE ANSWERS WITH RATIONALES

1. **d.** Health care facilities can have manual, computerized, or a combination of manual and computerized charge systems. (pages 129 and 131)

2. **c.** Health unit coordinators may receive a clinical or nonclinical shift report. (page 76)

3. **d.** A charge entered for patient equipment used on a daily basis is defined as a daily charge. (page 131)

4. **b.** A charge generated to the patient bill for goods, services, or equipment is defined as a patient charge. (page 126)

5. **a.** A purchase order is used when ordering supplies from an outside vendor. (page 128)

6. **a.** Patient acuity reflects the severity of the patient's condition and the level of care needed for the patient. (page 75)

7. **b.** The health unit coordinator is responsible for the upkeep of the patient census. (page 75)

8. **d.** The health unit coordinator can convey the hospital policy on visitor hours; all other visitor requests listed should be referred to the patient's nurse. (page 78)

9. **b.** Nursing care is the order classification for a treatment order. (page 394)

10. **b.** Diagnostic procedure is the order classification for a neurophysiology order. (page 394)

CHAPTER 9

Personnel Management

- ◆ Orient new staff members to the unit.

- ◆ Precept new or student unit coordinators.

- ◆ Communicate facility policies to visitors, patients, and staff (e.g., visiting hours, no smoking, etc.).

- ◆ Maintain staff assignment logs.

- ◆ Assist with unit staffing.

- ◆ Greet patients, physicians, visitors, and facility staff who arrive on the unit.

- ◆ Respond to patient, physician, visitor, and facility staff requests and complaints.

Recommended Reading

1. Read and review Chapters 15, 16, and 17 of *Health Unit Coordinator: 21st Century Professional*.

2. Read and review the key terms at the beginning of Chapters 15, 16, and 17 in *Health Unit Coordinator: 21st Century Professional*.

Key Terms

Andragogy a learner-focused approach to adult learning

Pedagogy the art of teaching children

CASE SCENARIO 1

Ali is a level-two certified health unit coordinator. She has attained a level-two status through her many years of excellent work ethic, certification, and assistance to all levels of staff on the nursing unit. Over the past 20 years, Ali has been the preceptor for four new health unit coordinators and about a dozen health unit coordinator interns (students) from the local vocational school, and she has trained numerous new nurses on their "desk orientation" day.

Years ago Ali attended a preceptor workshop offered by the nursing education department. She learned that a preceptor could be perceived to have three roles: to act as a role model—someone who serves as an example worthy of imitation; to act as an advocate—one who supports or helps another by defending or comforting; and to act as an educator—one who teaches or shares knowledge with another. She was also taught the principles of adult learning and the difference between andra-gogy, or a learner-focused approach to adult learning, and pedagogy, or the art of teaching children.

Ali always keeps a folder nearby that contains tools and some helpful hints she received in the workshop. Included in the folder are the four Knowles andragogical assumptions that:

1. Adults move from dependency to self-directedness
2. Adults draw upon their reservoir of experience for learning
3. Adults are ready to learn when they assume new roles
4. Adults want to solve problems and apply new knowledge immediately

Also included in the folder are: a copy of the hospital's mission (a written statement of purpose that defines the essence of the health care system) and vision statement (a written statement defining the health care system's future and the direction that will be pursued to achieve it); a current health unit coordinator job description; an orientation schedule; and an orientation checklist.

Something else that Ali took away from the workshop that she feels is very important—and yet she never had to write down—was the phrase "praise in public and criticize in private." She finds this to be extremely helpful when she is conducting orientations.

The role of the modern preceptor has become a little more challenging, and Ali may have to precept while also serving as the only health unit coordinator on the unit. This means that she must transcribe all orders, handle all communications, and coordinate all of the unit activities at the same time that she precepts a new health unit coordinator. However, Ali knows that this is all part of being a health unit coordinator that people respect. It is during the busy times like this that Ali must concentrate on her communication skills so that she can excel as a role model and be sure not to offend anyone. Ali uses numerous tools to help her keep organized and prepared to answer questions from new health unit coordinators, staff members, and visitors. These tools include bulletin boards, communication boards, and message boards.

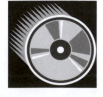

Case Scenario 1 Questions

1. Which of the following does not describe a preceptor?
   a. Role model
   b. Advocate
   c. Educator
   d. Coordinator

2. Which of the following best defines a vision statement?
   a. A written statement of purpose that defines the essence of the health care system
   b. A written statement defining the health care system's future and the direction that will be pursued to achieve it
   c. A written statement that defines the health care facility's customers
   d. A plaque to be seen by all who enter the health care facility

3. Which of the following best describes a tool to identify learning expectations?
   a. Orientation assessments
   b. Orientation checklists
   c. Job descriptions and competencies
   d. All of the above

4. It is best to praise in public and to criticize:
   a. Never
   b. Cautiously
   c. In public
   d. In private

5. Which of the following best defines an internship?
   a. A form of on-the-job training that usually combines job training with classroom instruction in trade schools, high schools, colleges, and universities
   b. A form of on-the-job training for medical students and physicians
   c. A form of on-the-job training that usually combines job training with classroom instruction only for colleges and universities
   d. All of the above

6. An educator is best defined as:
   a. One who teaches or shares knowledge with another
   b. One who does his or her job correctly
   c. One who serves as an example worthy of imitation
   d. All of the above

7. Which statement best describes a mission statement?

    a. A written statement of purpose that defines the essence of the health care system

    b. A written statement defining the health care system's future and the direction that will be pursued to achieve it

    c. A written statement that defines the health care facility's customers

    d. None of the above

8. A role model is best defined as:

    a. One who serves as an example worthy of imitation

    b. One who supports or helps another by defending or comforting

    c. One who teaches or shares knowledge with another

    d. All of the above

9. Andragogy is best defined as:

    a. A written statement defining the health care system's future and the direction that will be pursued to achieve it

    b. The art of teaching children

    c. A learner-focused approach to adult learning

    d. The study of preceptors

10. Which of the following is a tool used to assist the health unit coordinator in answering questions from staff and visitors?

    a. Communication boards

    b. Bulletin boards

    c. Message boards

    d. All of the above

CASE SCENARIO 2

Georgia, a certified health unit coordinator on an oncology unit at a regional university health system, was just finishing her shift. Georgia was venting to her manager, Tom, explaining that she was exhausted from all of the interpersonal actions she experienced during the day.

"Everyone must have woken up on the wrong side of the bed. The nurses, physicians, and visitors were grouchy and demanding. I felt like I couldn't do anything to please them. The admissions clerk told me she thought I was being rude when I didn't act happy enough for her when she called with the fourth admission this morning. Maybe I should go do a few cartwheels on her desk before I leave; do you think that will show her I love her admissions? And my favorite nurse, you-know-who, told anyone who would listen to take a look at all the unfinished orders piling up and that it never looks like this when Vanessa is the unit coordinator. I lost track of the times someone complained to me about having to wait for something. The phone calls were equally bad. A patient's wife actually cursed at me on the phone today. She said we were all a bunch of incompetent idiots. I can't even repeat the rest of what she said. All this because her transferred call was disconnected by mistake. For a moment, I wanted so badly to just hang up on her. I mean, I know she's going through a rough time, but I have feelings, too. Another caller wanted to know why we couldn't give them more details about her friend's condition. She said she was closer than a family member and that we were holding back information without reason. I mean, she was livid. I wanted to help, but it seemed like I was making matters worse. I don't think anyone really understands what it's like out here sometimes."

Tom tried to reassure Georgia: "No wonder you're stressed out; you had a lot going on. I hope you know I appreciate the work you do. Remember when you interviewed to transfer to this unit and we talked about the high stress level? I totally understand how crucial good communication skills are in your position. I'll make sure we have some time tomorrow to discuss this further and make sure you have the support you need. In the meantime, let me give you some information to review."

Later in the evening, Georgia read through the information her manager had given her and took some notes, as follows:

1. Understand your own reactions and responsibilities.

Think about your reactions to specific stressors or complaints. These could include reactions like "All he does is complain," "Why do I always have to work with her?" "He treats me unfairly," and "No one understands." These reactions turn your stressors into anger. It is important to recognize within yourself what turns your stressors or hurt into anger so you can avoid becoming defensive when dealing with angry complaints.

Accept your responsibility. When you decided to become a health unit coordinator, you also made the decision to serve people. When someone becomes angry and yells at you, you—and all others who work in the health care environment—lose your right to yell back. The customer deserves respect. Respect for people does not depend on accomplishments and is not diminished by bad behavior.

(continued)

It may be our job to handle complaints, but we have the right to be treated civilly and to not be subjected to abusive language. If the angry person resorts to obscene language, it is appropriate to set limits explaining that you cannot help if he or she continues to use foul language. If the angry person continues, let him or her know that you are going to end the conversation and will talk with the person when he or she can use better language.

2. Be an active listener.

Give the angry person your full attention; this means not allowing any distractions or trying to do other work while listening. Be polite and controlled. Use verbal and nonverbal communication to show interest and concern.

Ask the person to explain what happened and quietly wait for the answer. Give him or her at least a few minutes to talk without asking questions, interrupting, or offering a solution. Allow the person to vent. Take notes and write down any key issues that are brought to your attention.

It's hard to listen quietly to an angry person. Resist the temptation to interrupt or offer a solution before the person is finished. When he or she is finished, ask open-ended questions for clarification, such as "What day of the week did this occur?"

Don't become defensive, and don't take it personally. Even if the anger is being directed at you, you are not the source of the anger. Focusing on the facts may help you control your emotions. Realize that the angry person is trying to express a need; he or she is just going about it the wrong way at the moment.

3. Repeat what you think you have heard.

Repeat the complaint or concern as you understand it. State the need that you heard and let the person validate the information.

Acknowledge the difficulty the person experienced, and express empathy. It is not an admission of guilt to say that you are sorry the person had a difficult time. Let him or her know that you are trying to understand the problem.

4. Take action.

Let the person know that his or her concern has been heard and that you promise to do something to help. If there is something you can do, convey what it is and when you will do it. If the problem is out of your range of control, connect him or her with the appropriate resources. Use consultants in your facility, such as a psychiatric liaison nurse, guest advocate, social worker, psychologist, or chaplain. Be sure the resource is available before handing the angry person off to someone else.

The next day, Georgia's manager arranged to staff the workstation for an hour so that he and Georgia could talk. Georgia showed Tom her notes and was feeling more confident about how to handle the anger and stress she sometimes encounters on the job. Tom reviewed some of the health system's resources, such as the guest advocate department. Tom suggested that he and Georgia review some of the previous day's incidents and develop an alternative response based on what they had learned.

Case Scenario 2 Questions

1. Write a response from Georgia to the admissions clerk who told her she was being rude. Explain the response.

2. Write a response from Georgia to the nurse who compared her to the other coordinator. Explain the response.

3. Write a response from Georgia to the angry caller who cursed at her. Explain the response.

4. Write a response from Georgia to the angry caller who thought she was withholding information. Explain the response.

Fill in the Blank

Effective communication

Noise and activity

Receiver

Culture

Education level

Organizational culture

Reality shock

1. _____ _____ _____ affect communication, particularly when it may be difficult to hear as a result of activity in the area.

2. _____ affects communication when a person is dealing with many different ethnicities.

3. _____ _____ affects communication with regard to vocabulary used.

4. The _____ affects communication, especially when the communication is not face-to-face.

5. _____ _____ means the receiver receives the message and sends feedback to the sender.

Crossword Puzzle: Personnel Management

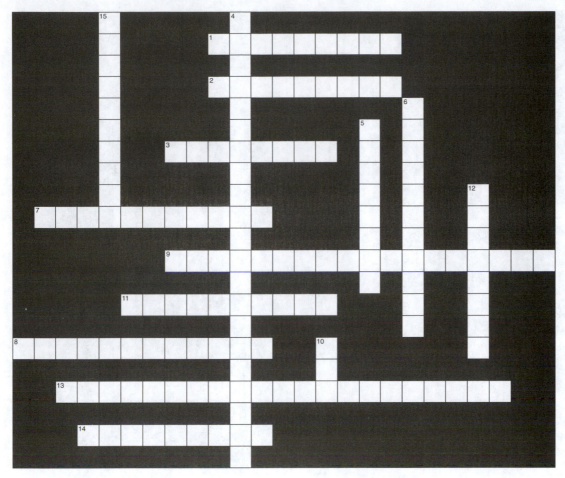

ACROSS

1. A learner-focused approach to adult learning
2. The stage in which a new hire may have the impression that everything is great
3. The art of teaching children
7. The planned introduction of new employees to their jobs, their coworkers, and the organization
8. The reaction that trainees have when they discover that the new work environment does not match the situation they had anticipated
9. A board used to communicate information to others
11. A form of on-the-job training that usually combines job training with classroom instructions in trade schools, high schools, colleges, and universities
13. A pattern of shared values and beliefs that gives members of an organization meaning and provides them with rules for behavior
14. An employee assigned to act as a role model, advocate, and educator for someone who is learning a new job responsibility

DOWN

4. Communication that is not planned
5. One who supports or helps another by defending or comforting
6. The customs or culture of a department
10. Personal digital assistant
12. The stage of reality shock in which the trainee is able to view the situation with a balanced perspective
15. A machine used to send and receive written materials from one place to another

■ CROSSWORD PUZZLE ANSWER

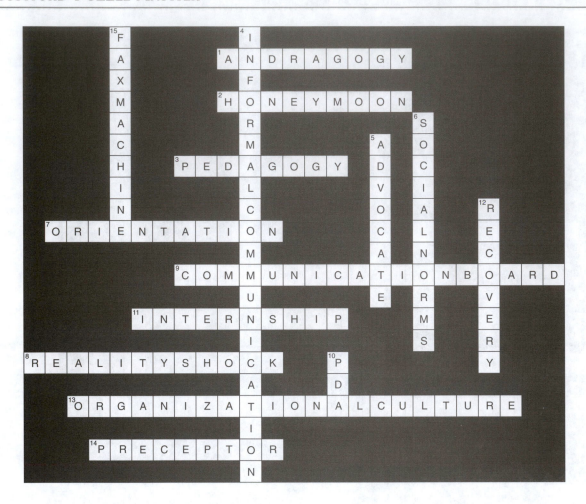

■ CASE SCENARIO 1 ANSWERS

1. **d.** A *preceptor* is best described as one who is a role model, advocate, and educator. (page 286)

2. **b.** A *vision statement* is a written statement defining the health care system's future and the direction that will be pursued to achieve it. (page 282)

3. **d.** Tools to identify learning expectations include orientation assessments, orientation checklists, and job descriptions and competencies. (page 290)

4. **d.** It is best to praise in public and criticize in private. (page 294)

5. **a.** An *internship* is a form of on-the-job training that usually combines job training with classroom instruction in trade schools, high schools, colleges, and universities. (page 281)

6. **a.** An *educator* is best defined as one who teaches or shares knowledge with another. (page 281)

7. **a.** A *mission statement* is a written statement of purpose that defines the essence of the health care system. (page 282)

8. **a.** A *role model* is best defined as one who serves as an example worthy of imitation. (page 282)

9. **c.** *Andragogy* is best defined as a learner-focused approach to adult learning. (page 290)

10. **d.** Tools that can assist the health unit coordinator in answering questions from staff and visitors are communication boards, bulletin boards, and message boards. (pages 276, 278, and 256)

■ CASE SCENARIO 2 SUGGESTED ANSWERS

1. Georgia could say, "I am sorry if you thought I was being rude. May I repeat back to you the information about this admission so I can be sure to set it up correctly?" Georgia could step back and admit to herself that she was stressed out about another admission and that her stress may have changed her tone of voice. She could simply say she was sorry and turn the focus back to the facts of the call.

2. Georgia could choose to ignore the comment or say, "This is not the first time you've compared me to Vanessa. Can we discuss this further privately, when we each have a free moment?" Georgia could realize that the nurse's comment made her angry because it hurt her to be compared to someone else and to have other people hear the comparison. She could choose to ignore the petty remark or address it in order to have a better working relationship with the nurse.

3. Georgia could say, "I am sorry you are upset. I want to help you. I cannot help you if you continue to curse at me. Please explain to me what happened without the cursing. If you continue to curse, I will ask you to call back when you can explain the problem without obscenities." Georgia does not have to tolerate the angry curses after she has stated her plan of action. She can ask for respect in order to be able to help.

4. Georgia could say, "Please explain to me what happened. I would like to know more about what upset you so I can help." After giving the caller time to explain, Georgia could repeat back the main complaint as she understands it. Since the complaint is about releasing information, Georgia would likely refer the complaint to the patient's nurse or nurse manager. Georgia should explain fully what she is going to do and what the expected time frame will be for a response.

■ FILL IN THE BLANK ANSWERS

1. Noise and activity
2. Culture
3. Education level
4. Receiver
5. Effective communication

References

Berger, B. A. (1998, August). Building effective relationships with your patients. *U.S. Pharmacist*, 52–64.

Reich, W. R. (1996). What care can mean for pharmaceutical ethics. *Journal of Pharmacy Teaching, 5*, 1–17.

CHAPTER 10

Safety and Security

- ◆ Maintain a hazard-free work environment.

- ◆ Maintain unit security.

- ◆ Participate in emergency and disaster plans.

- ◆ Respond to cardiac or respiratory arrests.

- ◆ Initiate call to cardiac or respiratory arrests.

- ◆ Comply with regulatory agency guidelines/rules.

Recommended Reading

Read and review Chapters 10 and 18 of *Health Unit Coordinator: 21st Century Professional.*

Abbreviations

MKAT   mandatory knowledge assessment tool

SDC   staff development coordinator

VCS   voice communication system

Key Terms

In-service   a meeting in which educational information is provided to the attendees

Safety manual   a book that contains all of the written policies and procedures for emergency situations in the health care facility

CASE SCENARIO

Ina has been a certified health unit coordinator on 4 West for the past four years. Tomorrow, at the unit staff meeting, the staff development coordinator (SDC) from education services will be at the unit in-service to review the mandatory knowledge assessment tool (MKAT). Every year, the staff must complete modules and review specific information to maintain the requirements established by the regulatory agencies for health care facilities. Ina wants to be prepared, so she plans to review the information prior to the in-service. Ina first reviews the safety manual—specifically the health unit coordinator's role in each emergency situation. The following is what she writes on her sheet to review later in the day:

Code 5—Cardiac Arrest: Dial 5, report the location, identify who you are, start CPR on the patient

Code Pink—Baby Abduction: Check the stairwells, look for anyone/anything unusual, report it to command center via voice communication system (VCS)

Code Red—Evacuation: Assist with moving patients to safe areas

Code 100—Fire: Close all open doors, help clear hallways, stay at workstation

Code 200—Bomb Threat: Stay at workstation, man the telephones

Code D—Disaster: Report to conference room #4 for instructions

Ina knows that on her unit last week there were three Code 5s, and that it is important for all of the health care team members know their role in emergency situations because there is a limited amount of time to do the right thing. As Ina puts the safety manual back on the shelf at the workstation, she hears the overhead paging system announce "Code 100 North Building 5th Floor" three times in a row. Ina quickly closes the door to the nourishment station and moves a w/c into the closet on her right. She then goes to the workstation and awaits future information.

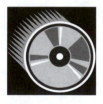

Case Scenario Questions

Unscramble the following words and place them in the sentences below to make each sentence true.

eltiaslwr

ttrkoswioan

riaccad

erhet

vi-ierscn

dre

aytsfe

tdasires

mregyeecn

dtnbcoaui

1. A Code 5 is a _____ arrest.

2. Ina will be attending a(n) _____ tomorrow to review the MKAT.

3. The _____ manual is where Ina finds the information she needs to know regarding her responsibility in specific code situations.

4. The overhead paging system announces the emergency code _____ times.

5. During a Code 200, Ina stays at the _____.

6. During a _____ Code, Ina reports to a specific conference room for instructions.

7. In a(n) _____ situation, there is limited time to respond.

8. Evacuation is a Code _____.

9. Code Pink is a baby _____.

10. During a Code Pink, the health unit coordinator on 4 West checks the _____.

Multiple Choice Questions

1. _____ is the science of fitting the job environment and equipment to the worker.
   a. Medicine
   b. Therapy
   c. Ergonomics
   d. Security

2. A(n) _____ contains information about types of chemicals and how to protect oneself from the risks of using the chemicals.
   a. MSDS
   b. SADS
   c. MDSS
   d. DASF

3. A(n) _____ report is a document used to record any event that resulted, or could have resulted, in injury or loss.
   a. safety
   b. incident
   c. medical
   d. patient

4. A(n) _____ agency is the term given to any agency outside the health care system that controls and monitors health and safety.
   a. government
   b. security
   c. regulatory
   d. none of the above

5. A special cart that contains _____ equipment is used in emergency situations; this may also be called a crash cart.
   a. fire
   b. life-saving
   c. disaster
   d. newborn

6. Departments that serve infants and children have a _____ policy in place, due to the chance of abduction.
   a. nursing
   b. visiting
   c. security
   d. health

7. The use of _____ does not eliminate the need for hand hygiene.
   a. gloves
   b. gowns
   c. masks
   d. none of the above

8. A fire emergency occurs whenever fire or _____ is detected.
   a. water
   b. smoke
   c. mist
   d. wind

9. The central supply department is responsible for the _____ and sterilization of patient care equipment.
   a. heating
   b. charging
   c. disinfection
   d. removal

10. Many services and procedures in the health care facility are expected to be performed _____.
    a. tomorrow
    b. later
    c. whenever
    d. stat

CRITICAL THINKING EXERCISE

Emergency Situations

Call three local health care facilities and complete the chart below.

Record the emergency code term for:

Emergency	Facility 1	Facility 2	Facility 3
Fire			
Disaster			
Cardiac arrest			
Infant abduction			
Combative person			
Bomb threat			
Weather			

Record the health unit coordinator's responsibility when the following codes are called:

Emergency	Facility 1	Facility 2	Facility 3
Fire			
Disaster			
Cardiac arrest			
Infant abduction			
Combative person			
Bomb threat			
Weather			

■ CASE SCENARIO ANSWERS

1. cardiac arrest
2. in-service
3. safety
4. three
5. workstation
6. disaster
7. emergency
8. red
9. abduction
10. stairwell

■ MULTIPLE CHOICE ANSWERS WITH RATIONALES

1. **c.** *Ergonomics* is the science of fitting the job environment and equipment to the worker. (page 150)

2. **a.** An *MSDS* contains information about types of chemicals and how to protect oneself from the risks of using them. (page 148)

3. **b.** An *incident* report is a document used to record any event that resulted, or could have resulted, in injury or loss. (page 146)

4. **c.** A *regulatory* agency is the term given to any agency outside of the health care system that controls and monitors health and safety. (page 140)

5. **b.** A special cart that contains *life-saving* equipment is used in emergency situations; this may also be called a crash cart. (page 152)

6. **c.** Departments that serve infants and children have a *security* policy in place, due to the chance of abduction. (page 154)

7. **a.** The use of *gloves* does not eliminate the need for hand hygiene. (page 157)

8. **b.** A fire emergency occurs whenever fire or *smoke* is detected. (page 152)

9. **c.** The central supply department is responsible for the *disinfection* and sterilization of patient care items. (page 148)

10. **d.** Many services and procedures in the health care facility are expected to be performed *stat*. (page 151)

CHAPTER 11

Confidentiality and Patient Rights

- ◆ Screen telephone calls and visitor requests for patient information to protect patient confidentiality.

- ◆ Restrict access to patient information (e.g., charts, computer, etc.).

- ◆ Assist with advance directive documentation.

- ◆ Demonstrate knowledge of informed consent.

Recommended Reading

Read and review Chapters 11, 12, 25, and 30 of *Health Unit Coordinator: 21st Century Professional.*

Key Terms

Informed consent the patient gives permission for a procedure after receiving full explanation of the procedure, the purpose, the benefits and the risks

CASE SCENARIO

Cathy is a responsible certified health unit coordinator. She understands that she must be able to answer for her conduct and for the actions she takes while working as a health unit coordinator. Cathy is familiar with the term *respondeat superior*, which is Latin for "let the master answer." This phrase means that a person's employer may also be held responsible for that employee's actions; however, Cathy knows that this is only true if one is following the policies and procedures of the employer. Therefore, Cathy is diligent about keeping current with policies and procedures because she knows that she is ultimately responsible for her actions. Cathy realizes that one of her most important responsibilities is to maintain confidentiality. In addition, she must be familiar with the facility's policies on patient rights.

Cathy begins each shift by reminding herself of her commitment to protect patient confidentiality and to perform all of her duties ethically. One morning, as Cathy walks to the hospital from the parking lot, she notices one of her coworkers frantically waving at her. The coworker runs up to her and explains that he has to make an important phone call before reporting to work; he asks Cathy to punch his time card into the time clock so it won't look like he is late. Cathy explains that she is not able to punch in his time card.

Cathy boards a busy elevator to get to her unit, along with other employees and visitors. Cathy overhears an employee sharing how sad she was that one of her favorite patients had taken a turn for the worse and had to be transferred to the intensive care unit. Cathy gently nudges the employee and nods her head toward the sign in the elevator that reads "Remember where you are—patient confidentiality is important." The employee tells Cathy, "I didn't mention any names."

When Cathy arrives on the unit, things are relatively quiet. Cathy notices that the computer at her desk is unattended but logged in. Cathy asks if anyone is currently using the computer, and the staff at the workstation tell her no. Cathy also notices that there are report forms at the workstation in clear view of anyone who stops at the desk. Cathy proceeds with organizing her work area.

A respiratory therapist asks Cathy for a patient's chart. Cathy looks in the chart rack and is unable to find it. She looks around the workstation, the medication room, and the staff lounge. Next, Cathy looks in the patient's room for the chart. She notices that the patient's room is empty, so she goes back to her computer and checks the patient's electronic Kardex. Cathy sees that the patient is scheduled for an early-morning colonoscopy. Cathy calls the gastroenterology department to confirm that the patient and the patient's chart are there.

The phone rings, and Cathy answers it. On the line is someone who claims to be from a physician's office, stating that he needs the results from the patient's laboratory tests. Cathy is unfamiliar with the caller and notices that the physician's name he gave does not match the physician's name on the patient's chart. Cathy inquires further, and the caller says that the physician is a new doctor who has been consulted by the patient's physician.

The activity level in the workstation increases. Cathy notices someone she is not familiar with reading a patient's chart. Cathy says, "I'm the unit coordinator today.

(continued)

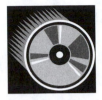

May I help you with something?" The individual responds, "No, thank you." Cathy notices that the individual is wearing scrub clothes and a stethoscope, but she is still unsure of the person's identity.

A visitor tells Cathy, "My father just told me he was having surgery today and he doesn't know why he has to have surgery." Cathy knows to check the chart for a form containing the patient's signature. Cathy locates the nurse who witnessed the form to talk with the family member. The nurse talks to the patient and family and then returns to Cathy to report that they now wish to talk to someone about the patient's wishes regarding life-sustaining treatment should he become irreversibly ill. Cathy calls the social services department to see if someone is available to assist the patient and family.

Case Scenario Questions

After reviewing the text and reading the case scenario, answer the following questions.

1. Cathy can be sure that her employer will take full responsibility for all of her actions on the job. Is this statement true or false? Explain why.

2. Many policies exist within the health care facility, and Cathy's manager will let her know which ones she needs to know. Is this statement true or false? Explain why.

3. Cathy has a moral duty to help out her coworker and punch his time card for him. Is this statement true or false? Explain why.

4. The employee in the elevator did not breach confidentiality because she did not mention any names. Is this statement true or false? Explain why.

5. The employee in the elevator did not breach confidentiality because her words showed that she truly cared about the patient. Is this statement true or false? Explain why.

6. Cathy should make sure that the unattended computer is logged off and then log back in with her own personal password. Is this statement true or false? Explain why.

7. Cathy should make sure that patient information—including laboratory reports—is not in plain sight of passersby. Is this statement true or false? Explain why.

8. What actions should have been taken when the patient and chart went to the gastroenterology department to ensure that the health unit coordinator would know the location of the patient and chart?

9. Cathy should answer the caller's request for laboratory results. Is this statement true or false? Explain why.

10. What actions could Cathy take with regard to the unfamiliar person reading the patient's chart?

11. What is the name of the form that Cathy checks to see if the surgery has been explained to the patient?

12. A living will explains who has been named to make health care decisions for the patient. Is this statement true or false? Explain why.

13. In Cathy's facility, social services assists the patient and family with advance directives. Is this statement true or false? Explain why.

Multiple Choice Questions

1. What does the unit coordinator do as the custodian of the patient's chart?

    a. Cleans the chart

    b. Hides the chart

    c. Protects the chart

    d. None of the above

2. It is good practice to refer phone calls from family members to the:

    a. Lead health unit coordinator

    b. Nurse caring for the patient

    c. Patient

    d. Physician

3. How many key areas are addressed in the HIPAA privacy act?

    a. 4

    b. 7

    c. 10

    d. 13

4. When the unit coordinator sees an unfamiliar person looking at a patient's chart, he or she should:

    a. Report it to the nurse manager

    b. Report it to the patient

    c. Determine the person's identity

    d. Do nothing; anyone with access to the workstation may view patient charts

5. What action can prevent unauthorized users from accessing patient information via the workstation computer?

    a. Lock the keyboard when leaving the computer unattended

    b. Log off when leaving the computer unattended

    c. Turn off the computer when leaving the computer unattended

    d. All of the above

6. Patient information may only be discussed with:

    a. Employees who are involved in the care of the patient

    b. Employees within the facility

    c. Employees with an employee photo identification badge

    d. Employees who can verify the patient's medical record number

7. Before surgery, the patient signs a consent form that contains the procedure name and a statement about which of the following?

    a. That the procedure and its risks have been explained

    b. That the physician is released from all responsibility

    c. Both a and b

    d. None of the above

8. A patient asks the health care provider to telephone test results directly to him or her at the patient's home phone number, and not to leave a message. Under which key area of the HIPAA privacy act is this covered?

    a. Access to medical records

    b. Prohibition of marketing

    c. Confidential communications

    d. Complaints

9. Generally, which type of procedure requires a signed consent form from the patient?

    a. Surgical procedure

    b. Dangerous procedure

    c. Experimental procedure

    d. Invasive procedure

10. Which of the following is a type of advance directive?

    a. Medical power of attorney

    b. Living will

    c. Patients' Bill of Rights

    d. Both a and b

Matching

Match the term in the left column with the definition in the right column.

_____ 1. Confidentiality

_____ 2. Ethical

_____ 3. HIPAA

_____ 4. PHI

_____ 5. Responsibility

_____ 6. Informed consent

_____ 7. Living will

_____ 8. Medical power of attorney

_____ 9. Due care

_____ 10. Liable

a. Obligated according to law

b. Conforming to a proper professional behavior

c. An act to provide continuous insurance coverage; includes privacy rules

d. The act of not providing certain information to anyone but another authorized person

e. The means by which an individual may appoint another person to make decisions about health care needs

f. Being able to answer for one's conduct and obligations

g. The duty to have adequate regard for another person's rights

h. The means by which an individual may express his or her wishes about life-sustaining treatment if he or she should become terminally ill

i. Private health information

j. Permission given after full disclosure of the facts

CRITICAL THINKING EXERCISE

HIPAA

Take this worksheet to a computer that has Internet capabilities and access the HIPAA Rules and Regulations from http://www.hhs.gov/ocr/hipaa/. In your own words, write at least three paragraphs on what you learned about the privacy rules after reviewing the site.

_____

_____

_____

_____

_____

_____

_____

_____

_____

_____

_____

_____

_____

_____

_____

_____

_____

_____

_____

_____

■ CASE SCENARIO SUGGESTED ANSWERS

1. This statement is false because the employer may be responsible for the employee's actions only if the employee is following the policies and procedures of the employer.

2. This statement is false because every employee is responsible for himself or herself.

3. This statement is false because punching someone else's time card is dishonest.

4. This statement is false because even if a name is not mentioned, confidentiality may be breached by the other information in the conversation.

5. This statement is false because patient information should always be protected even if it is positive or caring.

6. This statement is true because it ensures that all of the work Cathy enters into the computer is done only under her password.

7. This statement is true because Cathy should correct any possible breach of confidentiality she notices.

8. The transporter should have noted when the patient was removed from his or her room.

9. This statement is false because Cathy should not give the laboratory results over the phone until she confirms the identity of the person on the phone and checks the chart and/or Kardex to see if the physician is on the patient's case.

10. Cathy should confirm the identity of the person reading the chart. She could check with another staff person or ask the person directly.

11. The form that Cathy checks to see if the patient has signed to confirm that the surgery has been explained is titled *informed consent*.

12. This statement is false. Power of attorney explains who has been named to make health care decisions for the patient. A living will documents the patient's preference regarding life-sustaining procedures in the event of an irreversible illness.

13. This statement is true because Cathy contacts social services for the family when they wish to talk to someone about the patient's wishes regarding life-sustaining treatment should he become irreversibly ill. In other words, they wish to talk about a living will, which is a type of advance directive.

■ MULTIPLE CHOICE ANSWERS WITH RATIONALES

1. **c.** As custodian of the patient's chart, the unit coordinator protects it. (page 165)

2. **b.** It is good practice to refer phone calls from family members to the nurse who is caring for the patient. (page 169)

3. **b.** Seven key areas are addressed in the HIPAA privacy act. (page 126)

4. **c.** When the health unit coordinator sees an unfamiliar person looking at a patient's chart, he or she should determine the identity of that person. (page 165)

5. **b.** Logging off of the computer when leaving it unattended can prevent unauthorized users from accessing patient information via the workstation computer. (page 169)

6. **a.** Patient information may only be discussed with employees who are involved in the care of the patient. (page 165)

7. **a.** Before surgery, the patient signs a consent form that contains the procedure name and a statement that the procedure and its risks have been explained. (page 552)

8. **c.** When a patient asks the health care provider to telephone test results directly to him or her at the patient's home phone number and not to leave a message, this is covered under the confidential communications section of the HIPAA privacy act. (page 170)

9. **d.** Invasive procedures require a signed consent form from the patient. (page 437)

10. **d.** Both a medical power of attorney and a living will are examples of an advance directive. (page 177)

■ MATCHING ANSWERS

1. **d.** (page 162)
2. **b.** (page 163)
3. **c.** (page 170)
4. **i.** (page 163)
5. **f.** (page 163)
6. **j.** (page 552)
7. **h.** (page 176)
8. **e.** (page 176)
9. **g.** (page 162)
10. **a.** (page 163)

SECTION 3

Equipment/ Technical Procedures

CHAPTER 12

Communication

PART A Communicate with Patients and Staff via Intercom

- ◆ Review nonverbal communication skills.

- ◆ Review use of patient intercom system.

- ◆ Review facility- and department-specific policies and procedures regarding the use of communication devices.

Recommended Reading

Read and review Chapters 5, 15, and 16 of *Health Unit Coordinator: 21st Century Professional*.

Abbreviations

I/C   intercom

P&P   policy and procedure

Key Terms

Beeper or pager   an electronic device used to receive messages from another person; the device may be activated by phone to deliver a written or verbal message

Intercom   a device used to verbally communicate with another person usually not in physical view, such as communicating from a central location (e.g., the workstation) to another location (e.g., a patient room)

Intercom system   a system used to verbally communicate with a health care team member at the unit workstation or in other designated areas; also referred to as a *room call system* in Chapter 16

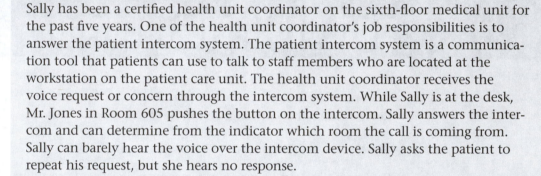

$\mathcal{C}$ASE SCENARIO

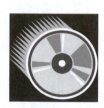

Sally has been a certified health unit coordinator on the sixth-floor medical unit for the past five years. One of the health unit coordinator's job responsibilities is to answer the patient intercom system. The patient intercom system is a communication tool that patients can use to talk to staff members who are located at the workstation on the patient care unit. The health unit coordinator receives the voice request or concern through the intercom system. While Sally is at the desk, Mr. Jones in Room 605 pushes the button on the intercom. Sally answers the intercom and can determine from the indicator which room the call is coming from. Sally can barely hear the voice over the intercom device. Sally asks the patient to repeat his request, but she hears no response.

Case Scenario Questions

Imagine you are Sally. What would you do next? Write down your next step and explain why you would take that action. Detail your steps according to your health system policy for this example.

_____

_____

_____

_____

_____

_____

Imagine you are the other health unit coordinator at the workstation while Sally is answering the intercom. What would you do next? Detail your steps according to your health system policy for this example.

_____

_____

_____

_____

_____

_____

Multiple Choice Questions

1. Nonverbal communication can be communicated via:
   a. Eye contact
   b. Words
   c. Voice
   d. Sound

2. Intercom devices used by patients are usually located in the:
   a. Patient's room, at his or her bedside
   b. Hallway
   c. Lounge
   d. Cafeteria

3. The intercom system in the patient's room is used routinely by the:
   a. Patient
   b. Housekeepers
   c. Physicians
   d. Lab assistants

4. A communication device is used to communicate information to the:
   a. Sender
   b. Receiver
   c. Middle man
   d. Neighbor

5. Which of the following is the most widely used communication device?
   a. Fax machine
   b. Beeper
   c. Telephone
   d. Pneumatic tube

6. The person using the patient intercom can detect a smile by the _____ of the speaker's voice.
   a. tone
   b. pitch
   c. pauses
   d. all of the above

7. Intercom systems allow patient concerns to be quickly communicated to:
   a. Family members
   b. Housekeeping
   c. Patient care providers at the workstation
   d. Physicians

8. Intercom systems save patient care providers _____ and provide quick responses to patient concerns.
   a. time
   b. money
   c. materials
   d. food

9. An intercom system allows the health unit coordinator to:
   a. Communicate with the patient
   b. Feel the patient
   c. See the patient's medical records
   d. View the patient's current medication list

10. As a health unit coordinator at the workstation, you can communicate quickly and conveniently with a patient using:
    a. Your personal cell phone
    b. Electronic mail
    c. The patient intercom system
    d. The fax machine

CRITICAL THINKING EXERCISE

Communication Devices

Use the following tear-out worksheet for this activity. Visit a workstation on a patient care unit to complete the exercises below. (Call and request through the nurse manager a four-hour block of time during which you can observe the health unit coordinator at the workstation.)

1. List at least six communication devices used at the workstation.

   _____

   _____

2. During a two-hour block of time, document how often the following communication devices are used by the health unit coordinator.

   Telephone:

   _____

   _____

   Fax machine:

   _____

   _____

   Patient intercom system:

   _____

   _____

3. List five items that patients request via the intercom system during your observation time at the workstation.

   _____

   _____

4. Locate the policy or procedure that addresses the use of communication devices. Summarize the information below, addressing the use of the intercom system.

   _____

   _____

■ MULTIPLE CHOICE ANSWERS WITH RATIONALES

1. **a.** Nonverbal communication can be communicated via *eye contact*. (page 253)

2. **a.** Intercom devices used by patients are usually located in the *patient's room, at his or her bedside*. (page 275)

3. **a.** The intercom system in the patient's room is used routinely by the *patient*. (page 275)

4. **b.** A communication device is used to communicate information to the *receiver*. (page 263)

5. **c.** The most widely used communication device is the *telephone*. (page 263)

6. **d.** The person using the patient intercom can detect a smile by the *tone, pauses,* and *pitch* of the speaker's voice. (page 265)

7. **c.** Intercom systems allow patient concerns to be quickly communicated to *patient care providers at the workstation*. (page 275)

8. **a.** Intercom systems save patient care providers *time* and provide quick responses to patient concerns. (page 276)

9. **a.** An intercom system allows the health unit coordinator to *communicate with the patient*. (page 275)

10. **c.** As a health unit coordinator at the workstation, you can communicate quickly and conveniently with a patient using *the patient intercom system*. (page 276)

■ CRITICAL THINKING POSSIBLE ANSWERS

1. Telephone, computer, fax machine, answering machine, room intercom system, overhead paging system, and beepers.

2. Telephone: 36 times

   Fax machine: 3 times

   Patient intercom system: 4 times

3. Assistance with personal needs, beverages and food, help to answer a phone call, pain medications, and to request a patient care provider.

4. Communication devices are to be responded to as quickly as possible, the intercom is to be answered immediately, and the nurse responsible for the patient's care is to be beeped right away with the patient's request, if applicable.

PART B Send and Receive Documents via Fax Machine

◆ Review written communication skills.

◆ Review use of the fax machine.

◆ Review facility- and department-specific policies and procedures regarding the use of fax communication.

Recommended Reading

Read and review Chapters 5, 15, and 16 of *Health Unit Coordinator: 21st Century Professional.*

Abbreviations

FBC   family birthing center

Key Terms

Confidentiality notice   a notice that states the intended use of a faxed document, including the confidentiality disclaimer

Cover sheet   a written document that contains information about the other faxed documents, including a disclaimer

Disclaimer   a written document stating that the information received is for the intended recipient only; if the actual recipient is not the intended recipient, the directions in the disclaimer should be followed

CASE SCENARIO

Susie, the certified health unit coordinator on the family birthing center (FBC) unit, has been busy transcribing physician orders all morning. She has one new patient admission—Mrs. Green—and two other patients—Mrs. Brown and Mrs. Bleau—who are being discharged in the afternoon. The new admission, Mrs. Green, is in Room 502; she needs to have an antibiotic started ASAP. Susie knows that the usual method of acquiring medications for new patients will take more than two hours. However, the medication needs to be given to Mrs. Green before then. Susie faxes the order for the medication to the pharmacy, and the pharmacy sends the correct medication to the unit in less than 15 minutes.

The two patients who are being discharged in the afternoon also have some special needs. Mrs. Brown in Room 503 needs to have a crib delivered to her home prior to taking home her new baby. Susie faxes the request to the local home equipment company. Before she sends the fax, Susie calls the company to make sure that she has the correct fax number and that the crib is available.

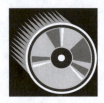

Mrs. Bleau in Room 502 will need a home health nurse to stop by once a day for a week to provide continuing nursing care for herself and her new baby. The social worker completes the required referral form, and Susie faxes this referral form to the home health agency that Mrs. Bleau has chosen. The home health agency will be better prepared to provide services to Mrs. Bleau and her baby when they receive the written information prior to visiting Mrs. Bleau at home the following morning.

Case Scenario Questions

1. Faxing orders to the pharmacy usually means that the medications will be sent to the patient unit faster than if orders are sent to the pharmacy the usual way.
   a. True
   b. False

2. Faxing orders to an agency prior to patient discharge allows the agency to be better prepared to provide the requested care to the patient.
   a. True
   b. False

3. A disclaimer form should never be sent with a fax.
   a. True
   b. False

4. Susie calls an off-site agency to make sure that the nurse is working that day.
   a. True
   b. False

5. All new patients on the unit have their orders faxed to the pharmacy.
   a. True
   b. False

6. The turnaround time for orders faxed to the pharmacy at the health care facility is more than two hours.
   a. True
   b. False

7. The equipment company is called to make sure that the special equipment is available prior to the order being faxed.
   a. True
   b. False

8. The home health agency receives a referral form completed by the unit clerk.
   a. True
   b. False

9. Susie has access to a fax machine.
   a. True
   b. False

10. Faxing is a method that may be used to provide better service to patients.
    a. True
    b. False

CRITICAL THINKING EXERCISE

Word Scramble

Unscramble the following words and write them in the correct spaces in the "Fill in the Blank" section that follows.

1. mdciilsare

2. ndsree

3. creedu

4. tunimse

5. trwitne

6. ssrue

7. crottpe

8. yiicpnhsa

9. ynmeo

10. teeerriv

Fill in the Blank

1. Faxed information should be preceded by a cover sheet that includes a _____.

2. The _____ should be notified if you receive an unintended fax.

3. Fax machines _____ errors.

4. Reports can be faxed to the offices of _____.

5. Fax machines copy _____ information that is fed into the machine.

6. Fax machines should be in areas that are easy for _____ to access.

7. Disclaimers _____ the senders.

8. Faxes save the patient time and _____.

9. If you are expecting a fax, you should be prepared to _____ it from the fax machine.

10. Information can be faxed within _____.

■ CASE SCENARIO ANSWERS

1. **a.** True
2. **a.** True
3. **b.** False
4. **b.** False
5. **b.** False
6. **b.** False
7. **a.** True
8. **b.** False
9. **a.** True
10. **a.** True

■ CRITICAL THINKING EXERCISE ANSWERS

1. disclaimer
2. sender
3. reduce
4. minutes
5. written
6. users
7. protect
8. physicians
9. money
10. retrieve

■ FILL IN THE BLANK ANSWERS WITH RATIONALES

1. Faxed information should be preceded by a cover sheet that includes a *disclaimer*. (page 270)
2. The *sender* should be notified if you receive an unintended fax. (page 271)
3. Fax machines *reduce* errors. (page 269)
4. Reports can be faxed to the offices of *physicians*. (page 270)
5. Fax machines copy *written* information that is fed into the machine. (page 269)
6. Fax machines should be in areas that are easy for *users* to access. (page 270)
7. Disclaimers *protect* the senders. (page 270)
8. Faxes save the patient time and *money*. (page 270)
9. If you are expecting a fax, you should be prepared to *retrieve* it from the fax machine. (page 270)
10. Information can be faxed within *minutes*. (page 269)

PART C Contact Personnel via Telecommunication Systems

◆ Review verbal communication skills.

◆ Review use of patient telecommunication systems.

Recommended Reading

Read and review Chapters 15 and 16 of *Health Unit Coordinator: 21st Century Professional.*

Abbreviation

Cell phone   cellular telephone

Key Terms

Beeps   an alert that is sent by the sender to a designated receiver device

Telecommunication   communication from a distance by electronic transmission

Telecommunication device   a piece of equipment that people use to communicate from a distance (e.g., telephone, fax machine, etc.)

Telecommunication systems   a network that people use to communicate with receiver(s) using an electronic communication device (e.g., hospital telephone systems)

Text message   typed communication into a telecommunication device that can be read by the receiver

CASE SCENARIO

Tom is a certified health unit coordinator working on the rehabilitation unit. At the workstation, Tom has a list of the current day's staff members and their corresponding telecommunication devices and numbers. Mrs. Jones, a patient in Room 804D, has just used the room call system to ask Tom if someone can come and help her get out of bed. Tom knows that Susie is the nursing assistant working with Mrs. Jones, so he checks the list and sees that Susie has cell phone #10, which is phone number 3410. Susie answers Tom, but she is busy helping out in Mr. Friend's room. Tom then beeps Gail and leaves a text message. Gail text messages back to Tom that she will go help Mrs. Jones. Gail knows how important it is to keep the nursing unit as quiet as possible; she had her beeper on silent mode but felt it vibrate when Tom beeped her. She was able to respond quickly and still keep the noise on the unit to a minimum. Tom didn't have to leave the workstation to look for the members of the patient care team because they were all connected through telecommunication devices, saving everyone time and providing faster customer service.

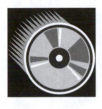

Case Scenario Questions

1. Tom had to leave the workstation to find the health care team members.
   a. True
   b. False

2. Telecommunication devices can save time.
   a. True
   b. False

3. The health unit coordinator must know how to use different telecommunication devices.
   a. True
   b. False

4. When telecommunication devices are used, they should be assigned to a specific staff member.
   a. True
   b. False

5. Text messaging is a quick way to communicate.
   a. True
   b. False

6. Telecommunication devices are always loud.
   a. True
   b. False

7. Keeping the nursing unit quiet was a priority for the staff.
   a. True
   b. False

8. Mrs. Jones used a cell phone to request help to get out of bed.
   a. True
   b. False

9. Providing good customer service is important to the members of this health care team.
   a. True
   b. False

10. Tom went to help Mrs. Jones.
    a. True
    b. False

Multiple Choice Questions

1. Verbal communication can be communicated via:
   a. Eye contact
   b. Touch
   c. Words
   d. Gestures

2. When a record of communication is required, the communication is:
   a. Written
   b. Nonverbal
   c. Passive
   d. Verbal

3. A(n) _____ can provide a message in voice or typed format.
   a. telephone
   b. beeper
   c. telefax machine
   d. intercom

4. Beeper alerts can be:
   a. Sounds
   b. Movements
   c. Flashes
   d. All of the above

5. The _____ is a handheld computer.
   a. fax machine
   b. PDA
   c. telephone
   d. pneumatic tube

6. The _____ _____ is an air-operated transport system.
   a. land phone
   b. cell phone
   c. pneumatic tube
   d. fax machine

7. E-mail is _____ mail.
   a. fast
   b. electronic
   c. business
   d. personal

8. _____ are used to store, process, send, receive, and retrieve information.
   a. Fax machines
   b. Telephones
   c. Computers
   d. Paging systems

9. _____ devices allow information to be communicated.
   a. Communication
   b. Data
   c. Physical
   d. Exercise

10. _____ communication can be formal or informal.
    a. Planned
    b. Direct
    c. Verbal
    d. Silent

CRITICAL THINKING EXERCISE

Telecommunication Devices

You will need to have a partner to complete this activity.

1. Conduct informal communication for two minutes. Have your partner write down three key points that were shared during the informal communication. Switch roles.

   _____

   _____

   _____

2. Using the three points that you each wrote down, present these points as formal communication to each other. Write the three key points as complete sentences with brief explanations. Limit length to one page.

   _____

   _____

   _____

3. Read the following sentence: *The pencil is here.* Speak this sentence to your partner a few times, changing your tone, loudness, and pauses each time. Switch roles. Discuss how changing the way you said the words changed the meaning of the sentence.

   _____

   _____

   _____

4. Demonstrate three nonverbal gestures that could be used in a health care setting. Write down the meanings of the gestures.

   _____

   _____

   _____

■ CASE SCENARIO ANSWERS

1. **b.** False
2. **a.** True
3. **a.** True
4. **a.** True
5. **a.** True
6. **b.** False
7. **a.** True
8. **b.** False
9. **a.** True
10. **b.** False

■ MULTIPLE CHOICE ANSWERS WITH RATIONALES

1. **c.** Verbal communication can be communicated via *words*. (page 251)
2. **a.** When a record of communication is required, the communication is *written*. (page 255)
3. **b.** A *beeper* can provide a message in voice or typed format. (page 269)
4. **d.** Beeper alerts can be *sounds, flashes,* or *movements*. (page 269)
5. **b.** The *PDA* is a handheld computer. (page 263)
6. **c.** The *pneumatic tube* is an air-operated transport system. (page 274)
7. **b.** E-mail is *electronic* mail. (page 273)
8. **c.** *Computers* are used to store, process, send, receive, and retrieve information. (page 270)
9. **a.** *Communication* devices allow information to be communicated. (page 263)
10. **c.** *Verbal* communication can be formal or informal. (page 251)

PART D Answer and Process Unit Telephone Calls

- ◆ Review telephone skills for the sender.
- ◆ Review telephone skills for the receiver.
- ◆ Discuss the importance of taking messages.

Recommended Reading

Read and review Chapters 15 and 16 of *Health Unit Coordinator: 21st Century Professional.*

Abbreviations

D/T date and time

OPC outpatient cardiac

Key Terms

Answering machine a device that records a voice message that can be replayed in the future

Archives voice mail messages that can be stored for a specific amount of time in a voice mail account

Voice mail a message that is recorded into an electronic device that can be replayed in the future on request

Voice mailbox an area housed in an electronic device that can be accessed by an individual to retrieve his or her oral messages; usually requires a password for access

CASE SCENARIO

Jenna is a certified health unit coordinator working on the outpatient cardiac (OPC) unit. She has four telephones at her workstation. Three of the telephones are connected to the hospital telephone system, and the fourth is a direct line to the outside telephone system. Two of the in-house telephones lines are ringing at the same time, and Jenna is the only staff person at the workstation. She answers the first line and asks if she can put the person on hold. She answers the second ringing line before the third ring and responds to the caller's request. The caller asks to speak to the nurse manager who is not on the unit today. Jenna asks the caller if she would like to leave a voice mail for the manager. Jenna then transfers the call into the voice mail system. She returns to the first caller and responds to his request to speak with his father, who is in Room 116. Jenna transfers the call to Room 116. She waits until the telephone is answered in Room 116, announces the caller, and then disconnects her telephone line from the call. The direct outside line is now ringing, and Jenna answers the call the same way she answers all telephone calls: by identifying her name, position, and location to the caller. Jenna answers using only her first name, which is the policy at her hospital. The caller is the home health nurse, who would like to leave a written message for Mr. Jones, the patient in Room 406D. Jenna writes down the message, reads it back to the caller, adds the date and time (D/T), and delivers it to Mr. Jones's nurse, who will bring the written message to him.

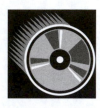

Case Scenario Questions

1. Jenna is able to direct callers to leave messages using _____ _____.

2. It is important to answer the telephone by the _____ ring, if possible.

3. You should always ask permission prior to putting a caller on _____.

4. Some people want to leave _____ messages for patients.

5. Telephone calls can be _____ into patient rooms.

6. Telephone calls come from people inside and _____ the hospital.

7. When answering the telephone, it is important to provide the caller with your name, _____, and location.

8. Jenna only providers her _____ name to the callers when she answers the telephone.

9. Sometimes, more than one _____ may ring at the same time.

10. It is important to make sure that the person to whom you are transferring a call answers the call prior to you _____ your telephone line.

Multiple Choice Questions

1. A _____ telephone is free of connecting lines.
   a. land
   b. cell
   c. box
   d. none of the above

2. The primary limitation of the cell phone is the need to _____ it.
   a. replace
   b. recharge
   c. reconnect
   d. reboot

3. You should only place a caller on _____ after you have asked permission.
   a. computer
   b. beeper
   c. hold
   d. intercom

4. Callers form a mental picture of the _____ even though they cannot see the person.
   a. operator
   b. nurse
   c. receiver
   d sender

5. The speaker's tone, _____, and pause can send a smile through telephone lines.
   a. pitch
   b. frown
   c. eyes
   d. language

6. Do not have _____ in your mouth when answering the telephone.
   a. food
   b. gum
   c. candy
   d. all of the above

7. It is important to project a _____ attitude to others on the telephone.
   a. normal
   b. bored
   c. positive
   d. negative

8. _____ are one of the most frequently used communication devices.
   a. Fax machines
   b. Telephones
   c. Computers
   d. Paging systems

9. Always end telephone calls with a(n) _____ _____.
   a. question mark
   b. information request
   c. thank you
   d. telephone number

10. First impressions are based on voice _____, voice tone, and interest level.
    a. volume
    b. pauses
    c. enunciation
    d. speed

CRITICAL THINKING EXERCISE

Telephones

1. Call your local hospital on the telephone and ask the operator to connect you to a nursing unit. Document the following:

   a. How many times did the telephone ring before it was answered?_____

   b. Were you asked to be put on hold?_____

   c. How was the telephone answered?

      i. Name-_____

      ii. Unit-_____

      iii. Position-_____

   d. Describe your mental picture of the person who answered the telephone based on what you heard and felt.

      _____

      _____

      _____

      _____

   e. How did the conversation end?

      _____

      _____

      _____

      _____

   If possible, repeat this exercise more than once. Compare your results.

■ CASE SCENARIO ANSWERS

1. voice mail
2. third
3. hold
4. written
5. transferred
6. outside
7. position
8. first
9. telephone
10. disconnecting

■ MULTIPLE CHOICE ANSWERS WITH RATIONALES

1. **b.** A *cell* telephone is free of connecting lines. (page 264)

2. **b.** The primary limitation of the cell phone is the need to *recharge* it. (page 264)

3. **c.** You should only place a caller on *hold* after you have asked permission. (page 265)

4. **c.** Callers form a mental picture of the *receiver* even though they cannot see the person. (page 265)

5. **a.** The speaker's tone, *pitch,* and pause can send a smile through the telephone lines. (page 263)

6. **d.** Do not have *food, gum,* or *candy* in your mouth when answering the telephone. (page 265)

7. **c.** It is important to project a *positive* attitude to others on the telephone. (page 267)

8. **b.** *Telephones* are one of the most frequently used communication devices. (page 267)

9. **c.** Always end telephone calls with a *thank you.* (page 267)

10. **a.** First impressions are based on voice *volume,* voice tone, and interest level. (page 267)

CHAPTER 13

Computers

- ◆ Maintain computer census (i.e., ADT functions).

- ◆ Retrieve diagnostic results from computers.

- ◆ Follow established computer downtime procedures.

- ◆ Enter orders via computer.

- ◆ Schedule appointments via computer.

- ◆ Prepare documents using computer software.

- ◆ Generate reports via computer.

- ◆ Operate computers safely and correctly.

- ◆ Troubleshoot problems with computers.

Recommended Reading

Read and review Chapters 16 and 31 of *Health Unit Coordinator: 21st Century Professional*.

Abbreviations

ADT   admission, discharge, and transfer

Biomed   biomedical electronics department

P&P   policy and procedures

CASE SCENARIO

David is a certified health unit coordinator supervisor at a regional acute care hospital. David's facility is the only full-service hospital that is available to patients for miles around. The hospital contains several types of inpatient units, such as medical, surgical, pediatrics, cardiac, neurology, oncology, orthopedic, mother and baby, and intensive care. There are approximately six full-time and part-time health unit coordinators employed on each of the inpatient units. David supervises the day-shift health unit coordinators on all of the units.

As their supervisor, David is responsible for covering for their absences and working on the units when necessary. Because David may be called to work on any of the units, he must have authorization to access each of the units' computers. The health information services gave David a password with full access to all of the computer programs for the inpatient hospital units.

As supervisor, David is also a resource person, and he receives calls from his staff when they have questions about the computers. He must know about both the software and the hardware. David's staff uses the order entry software the majority of the time, as well as the admission, discharge, and transfer (ADT) and test results functions. Some of his staff also use the office suite software, such as word processing, database management, and spreadsheets. David has created a help sheet that he carries with him to answer the most frequently asked questions. The information on David's help sheet is as follows:

Hardware Troubleshooting:

1. First, check all cord connections from the CPU to the monitor, the keyboard, the mouse, and the printer.
2. Second, check all electrical connections.
3. Third, refer to the computer troubleshooting section of the Biomedical Electronics Policy and Procedures (P&P) Manual.
4. If unable to resolve, contact biomedical electronics personnel via pager 45624.
5. If biomedical personnel do not answer the in-house pager within 20 minutes, contact biomedical electronics emergency on-call staff via pager (555) 555-5625.

Software Troubleshooting:

1. Select F1 from the menu for the order entry screen.
2. Select F2 from the menu to retrieve and print diagnostic test results.
3. Select F3 from the menu for ADT functions.
4. Select F4 from the menu to schedule appointments with regional clinic physicians.
5. Select F6 from the menu to access the link to the office suite software.
6. For order entry, ADT, results, and appointment functions, refer to the inpatient nursing unit section of the Information Systems P&P Manual.
7. For office suite software, refer to the manufacturer's user manuals.

(continued)

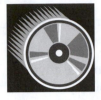

Downtime Procedure:

1. Inform staff of the downtime via overhead page and phone calls.

2. Obtain a supply of general paper requisitions from the print shop.

3. For downtimes of two hours or less, process stat orders only via paper requisition and phone. Paper requisitions may be sent to the appropriate departments via fax, pneumatic tube, or hand delivery. Copies of paper requisitions are to be kept at the workstation to be entered into the computer when the downtime is over.

4. For downtimes of more than two hours, process all orders via paper requisition and phone. Paper requisitions may be sent to the appropriate departments via fax, pneumatic tube, or hand delivery. Copies of paper requisitions are to be sent to the information systems department to be entered into the computer when the downtime is over.

Case Scenario Questions

Based on the information in the case scenario, answer the following questions.

1. Under which menu selection would one likely find information about the unit's census?

2. Under which menu selection would one likely retrieve laboratory results?

3. Under which menu selection would one likely schedule a doctor's appointment?

4. Under which menu selection would one likely print a radiology report?

5. Under which menu selection would one likely transfer a patient from a private room to a semiprivate room?

6. Under which menu selection would one likely request a low-sodium diet for a patient?

7. Who is responsible for entering orders after a downtime of five hours?

8. The staff is notified of information systems downtime via e-mail. Is this statement true or false?

9. Only stat orders are processed during a downtime that lasts one hour. Is this statement true or false?

10. All orders are processed during a downtime that lasts three hours. Is this statement true or false?

11. Where does David obtain paper requisitions?

12. David should be able to access the billing department's programs with the type of password he has. Is this statement true or false?

13. What should David use to best answer a question about spreadsheet software?

14. What should David use to best answer a question about how to discharge a patient in the system?

15. What should David use to best answer a question about how to order a bone scan?

16. David should be able to use the F4 menu selection to schedule an appointment with a physician from another hospital outside of the region. Is this statement true or false?

17. David should be able to use the F6 menu selection to access the word processing software. Is this statement true or false?

18. David receives a call from one of his staff members, who says he can't see anything on his computer screen; in response, David should first call biomedical personnel. Is this statement true or false?

19. David receives a call from one of his staff members, who says she can't get the order entry function to work correctly; in response, David should first ask her to check all of her cord connections. Is this statement true or false?

20. What should David do if he paged biomed 45 minutes ago and they haven't responded?

Multiple Choice Questions

1. What is used to ensure that the computer user has access only to the information and programs needed to do his or her job?

   a. Identification code and password

   b. Policy and procedures

   c. Locked keyboard and motherboard

   d. All of the above

2. What is the term given to a picture that is used to represent an object?

   a. HTML tag

   b. Hyperlink

   c. Icon

   d. Port

3. Which of the following is hardware that resembles a typewriter keypad?

   a. Computer brains

   b. Keyboard

   c. Monitor

   d. Number keypad

4. Which of the following is hardware that resembles a television screen?

   a. Computer brains

   b. Keyboard

   c. Monitor

   d. Files

5. What term is given to the hardware that stores components required for the computer to function?

   a. Computer brains/CPU

   b. Keyboard

   c. Monitor

   d. Files

6. Which of the following best defines a "network"?

   a. Computer systems that are stand-alone and work independently

   b. Computer systems that allow more than one workstation access to the same programs

   c. A satellite system that provides continuing education programming

   d. None of the above

7. What do computers do with information?

   a. Process it

   b. Send and receive it

   c. Store it

   d. All of the above

8. Which of the following might be used to shield visible information displayed on a computer screen?

   a. Screen protector

   b. Screen saver

   c. Screen encrypter

   d. All of the above

9. Which of the following is an alternate term that may be given to the cabinet that houses the internal computer devices that store programs and other components required for the computer to function?

   a. Tower

   b. Black box

   c. Obelisk

   d. Cubbyhole

10. Which of the following is an example of the types of computer programs that may be stored in the workstation computer?

    a. Word processing

    b. Database

    c. Supply tracking

    d. All of the above

Matching

Unscramble the information services key terms in the left column, and then match each one with its correct information systems definition in the right column.

_____ 1. Resrev

_____ 2. Yelrinhkp

_____ 3. Ximizema

_____ 4. Stakarb

_____ 5. Ficnterae

_____ 6. Rtop

_____ 7. Momed

_____ 8. Unem

_____ 9. Ddoownla

_____ 10. Llaco reaa tnekorw

a. The portion of the screen that includes the start button, the time display, and everything in between

b. A data communications system often confined to a limited geographical area with moderate to high data rates

c. To make a window take up a full screen

d. A place of access to a device or network, used for input and output of digital and analog signals

e. A computer that runs software that allows it to control the sharing of resources among other computers

f. Refers to a link imbedded in a document

g. To copy information from one computer to another

h. The connection between two computer components

i. A device that allows computers to communicate with one another over phone lines

j. A list of available functions

CRITICAL THINKING EXERCISE

Computers

Take this worksheet to a health care workstation. Ask an authorized staff person to show you the workstation computer equipment, along with the computer menu selections that are available to the health unit coordinator. Answer the following questions.

1. How many computer stations are there at the workstation or on the unit?

   _____

   _____

2. How many printers are there at the workstation or on the unit?

   _____

   _____

3. Where are the computer P&P manuals stored?

   _____

   _____

4. What are the titles of the computer P&P manuals?

   _____

   _____

5. Locate the downtime P&P. In your own words, explain the process.

   _____

   _____

   _____

   _____

6. List the menu selections that are used by health unit coordinators at the workstation.

   _____

   _____

■ CASE SCENARIO SUGGESTED ANSWERS

1. F3
2. F2
3. F4
4. F2
5. F3
6. F1
7. Information systems department
8. False
9. True
10. True
11. Print shop
12. False
13. Manufacturer's user manual
14. Information Systems Policy and Procedures Manual
15. Information Systems Policy and Procedures Manual
16. False
17. True
18. False
19. False
20. Contact the biomedical emergency on-call staff via pager

■ MULTIPLE CHOICE ANSWERS WITH RATIONALES

1. **a.** The combination of *identification code and password* is used to ensure that the computer user has access only to the information and programs needed to do his or her job. (page 273)
2. **c.** *Icon* is the term given to a picture that is used to represent an object. (page 566)
3. **b.** The *keyboard* is hardware that resembles a typewriter keypad. (page 272)
4. **c.** The *monitor* is hardware that resembles a television screen. (page 272)
5. **c.** *Computer brains/CPU* is the term given to the hardware that stores other components required for the computer to function. (page 272)
6. **b.** Networks are *computer systems that allow more than one workstation access to the same programs.* (page 273)
7. **d.** Computers *process, store, send, receive,* and *retrieve* information. (page 270)
8. **a.** A *screen saver* might be used to shield visible information displayed on a computer screen. (page 272)
9. **a.** When the computer cabinet is narrow and tall, it is commonly called a *tower*. (page 272)
10. **d.** *Word processing, database,* and *supply-use tracking* programs are all examples of the types of computer programs that may be stored in the workstation computer. (page 272)

■ MATCHING ANSWERS

1. **e.** Server
2. **f.** Hyperlink
3. **c.** Maximize
4. **a.** Taskbar
5. **h.** Interface
6. **d.** Port
7. **i.** Modem
8. **j.** Menu
9. **g.** Download
10. **b.** Local area network

CHAPTER 14

Monitoring System

- ◆ Register a patient into the monitoring system.
- ◆ Print and mount strips.

Recommended Reading

1. Read and review Chapters 13 and 25 of *Health Unit Coordinator: 21st Century Professional*.

2. Use a medical dictionary to assist you in answering the multiple-choice questions in this chapter.

Abbreviations

EP   electrophysiology

MBO   monitored bed orders

PTCA   percutaneous transluminal coronary angioplasty

Key Terms

Angiogram   an X-ray of one or more blood vessels that is produced by angiography and used to diagnose pathological conditions

Angioplasty   to reshape the blood vessel using a balloon to open obstructed arteries

Coronary   specifies that the coronary artery is being treated

Electrophysiology   the electric activity associated with a bodily part or function

Percutaneous   to access the blood vessel through the skin

Transluminal   a procedure performed within the blood vessel

CASE SCENARIO

Jane has worked as a certified health unit coordinator on the orthopedic unit for 10 years. She has recently transferred to a telemetry unit because of schedule preferences. Jane is aware that the orders will be different than those she has seen on the orthopedic unit. She knows patients will use telemetry, a monitoring system that measures and transmits heart activity. Jane's preceptor has shown her where the monitored bed orders (MBO) are kept for all patients on telemetry. Jane was also informed that the majority of patients on the unit are recovering from a cardiac catheterization, a percutanenous transluminal coronary angioplasty (PTCA), or an electrophysiology (EP) study.

When a new patient arrives, one of Jane's responsibilities will be to place specific patient data into the telemetry system by entering the patient's full name, medical unit number, financial number, and room location. Toward the end of the shift, the health unit coordinators are responsible for affixing the telemetry tracings that printed out during the shift onto a specific supplemental chart form—making sure the patient's name, date, and time of the tracing are legible—and then filing them into the patients' charts by the end of the shift.

Other health unit coordinator duties, such as computer order entry, chart maintenance, communication, and coordination of unit activities, are similar to those on the orthopedic unit.

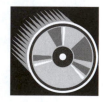

Case Scenario Questions

Indicate whether each of the following questions is true or false.

1. If a patient is on telemetry, the health unit coordinator needs to place MBO forms on his or her chart.

2. Jane's new responsibilities include computer order entry.

3. PTCA is the abbreviation for post transluminal coronary angiogram.

4. The physician's name must be included when a new patient's data is entered into the telemetry system.

5. Jane's new responsibilities include affixing the telemetry strips onto a supplement chart form.

6. Jane's new responsibilities will include transcribing PTCA orders.

7. Telemetry strips need to be read by a physician before they are filed in the patient's chart.

8. When filing the telemetry strips, Jane needs to ensure that the patient's birth date is legible.

9. When the telemetry strips are affixed, the patient's financial number must be legible.

10. When the telemetry strips are affixed, the patient's medical record unit number must be legible.

Multiple Choice Questions

1. What does the abbreviation EP stand for?
   a. Electrophysical therapy
   b. Electrophysiology
   c. Electrophysical studies
   d. Electrocardiogram

2. Which term is used for a procedure performed within the blood vessel?
   a. Percutaneous
   b. Coronary
   c. Transluminal
   d. Catheterization

3. Which term is used to specify that the coronary artery is being treated?
   a. Electrophysiology
   b. Angiogram
   c. Coronary
   d. Transluminal

4. Which of the following best describes a unique number that is assigned to a patient each time he or she is admitted to a health care facility?
   a. Account number
   b. Financial number
   c. Medical record number
   d. Both a and b

5. Which of the following best describes an X-ray of one or more blood vessels that is produced by angiography and used to diagnose pathological conditions?
   a. Angiogram
   b. Electrophysiology
   c. Coronary
   d. Percutaneous

6. What does the abbreviation MBO stand for?
   a. Monitored bed observation
   b. Monitored bed orders
   c. Monitored bio orders
   d. Mostly bed observation

7. What does the abbreviation PTCA stand for?
   a. Post transluminal coronary angiogram
   b. Post transluminal catheterization angiogram
   c. Percutaneous transluminal catheterization angiogram
   d. Percutaneous transluminal coronary angioplasty

8. A cardiac catheterization is best defined as:
   a. An invasive procedure in which a long catheter is passed into the heart through a large blood vessel in an arm or leg to diagnose heart disease
   b. A procedure performed within the blood vessel
   c. An X-ray of one or more blood vessels that is produced by angiography and used to diagnose pathological conditions
   d. All of the above

9. An ECG is best defined as which of the following?
   a. A noninvasive exam performed by a technician using sound frequencies to study the function of the heart
   b. A noninvasive exam that records electrical impulses of the heart
   c. A procedure performed within the blood vessel
   d. An invasive procedure in which a long catheter is passed into the heart through a large blood vessel in an arm or leg to diagnose heart disease

10. Which of the following best defines telemetry?
   a. A noninvasive exam performed by a technician using sound frequencies to study the function of the heart
   b. A procedure performed within the blood vessel
   c. A device that monitors heart activity throughout the course of the day
   d. The process of measuring and transmitting heart activity during hospitalization

CRITICAL THINKING EXERCISE

Using the Internet, search for "electrophysiology" to find more tests that are performed in an electrophysiology department. List four tests and a brief explanation of each one, including the necessary preparation.

_____

_____

_____

_____

_____

_____

_____

_____

_____

_____

_____

_____

_____

_____

_____

_____

_____

■ CASE SCENARIO ANSWERS

1. True
2. False
3. False
4. False
5. True
6. True
7. False
8. False
9. True
10. False

■ MULTIPLE CHOICE ANSWERS WITH RATIONALES

1. **b.** EP is the abbreviation for *electrophysiology*. (medical dictionary)

2. **c.** *Transluminal* refers to a procedure performed within the blood vessel. (medical dictionary)

3. **c.** *Coronary* is the term that specifies that the coronary artery is being treated. (medical dictionary)

4. **d.** The *account number* and the *financial number* are both unique numbers assigned to a patient each time he or she is admitted to a health care facility. (pages 187 and 188)

5. **a.** An *angiogram* is an X-ray of one or more blood vessels that is produced by angiography and used to diagnose pathological conditions. (medical dictionary)

6. **b.** MBO is the approved abbreviation for *monitored bed orders*. (page 436)

7. **d.** PTCA is the abbreviation for *percutaneous transluminal coronary angioplasty*. (medical dictionary)

8. **a.** A *cardiac catheterization* is best defined as an invasive procedure in which a long catheter is passed into the heart through a large blood vessel in an arm or leg to diagnose heart disease. (page 440)

9. **b.** An ECG is *a noninvasive exam that records electrical impulses of the heart*. (page 440)

10. **d.** *Telemetry* is best defined as the process of measuring and transmitting heart activity during hospitalization. (page 440)

CHAPTER 15

Miscellaneous Equipment

- ◆ Duplicate documents using a copy machine.
- ◆ Transport patient specimens, supplies, and medications using pneumatic tubes.

Recommended Reading

Read and review Chapters 5, 16, and 28 of *Health Unit Coordinator: 21st Century Professional.*

Abbreviations

AMD   automated medication dispensing

N/O   neuro/ortho

SCN   special care nursery

VCS   voice communication system

Key Terms

Automated medication dispensing device   a machine that is programmed to provide patient drugs when health care providers enter the correct information

Overhead page   a voice system that announces information throughout a specific area using microphones

Pet partners   a group of people who bring tame animals to visit patients

Voice communication system   more than one wireless device connected to other devices, allowing the users to talk to one another instantly

CASE SCENARIO

Lee, a certified health unit coordinator in the special care nursery (SCN), has been asked to work on the neuro/ortho (N/O) unit the following day. Lee has agreed to do so but asks if she can spend an hour with the health unit coordinator beforehand to familiarize herself with the workflow and equipment of the unit. Lee arrives on N/O at 2:00 P.M. and sees the following equipment:

1. telephones
2. computers
3. copier
4. fax machine
5. automated medication dispensing (AMD) machine
6. voice communication system (VCS) terminal
7. pneumatic tube terminal
8. padded and unpadded pneumatic tubes
9. scanner

Lee is familiar with some of the equipment, but not all of it. She asks the following questions so that she will be prepared to work the shift she has agreed to take. Joanna, who is the certified health unit coordinator Lee will be working for, answers each of her questions.

Question	Answer
1. What is the unit telephone number?	The unit telephone number is 376-4353.
2. What is the unit ID to enter into the computer programs? What programs do you have access to on this unit?	"Noor" is the unit ID. The unit accesses server GL and GQ for the patient care programs.
3. What is the password for the copier? And what do you use it for?	The password is 4353. We use the copier to photocopy information for the staff; patient information is not copied on this machine.
4. What is the fax number?	The fax number is 376-4354.
5. Do you fax or scan orders to the pharmacy?	We scan orders to our pharmacy and fax orders to outside pharmacies.
6. Does the health unit coordinator do anything with the AMD device?	The pharmacy exchanges the AMD device at 9:00 A.M.; the UC doesn't do anything with the device.

(continued)

7. What do you use the unpadded and padded tubes for, and where are they stored?	The unpadded tubes are used by the pharmacy to send stat drugs to the unit, and by other departments to send paper information to the unit. The padded tubes are only used to send blood samples to the lab; they are stored in the cupboard under the system.
8. How many tubes is your unit allowed to hold in the pneumatic tube storage area?	We are assigned four tubes; any more than that can be sent to 90.
9. What time do you tube your diet sheet to the dietary department?	The sheet is tubed at 11:00 A.M. for lunch.
10. Where is the VCS log? Does the UC assign the devices after report?	Yes, the devices are assigned by the UC, and the log is kept in the slot by the VCS machine.
11. Is there anything that I should be aware of that will take place tomorrow? Or that I will need to do?	Our admissions arrive usually at 10:00 A.M., and our discharges usually leave the unit by 9:00 A.M. Our ORs usually arrive after 3:00 P.M. On Wednesdays we have pet partners come to the patient lounge at 2:00 P.M. They will let you know when they arrive so that you can announce that information to the unit via overhead page.
12. Where is your communication book?	The communication book is kept by the telephone; I will write you a note if there is anything else that you should be aware of for tomorrow. Please leave me a note about anything that needs to be followed up on Thursday.

Lee makes notes of the answers that Joanna gives her and knows that she is prepared and ready to work the N/O unit the following day, now that she is familiar with the equipment and knows the workflow process.

Case Scenario Questions

Based on the information in the case scenario, answer the following questions.

1. The unit has a specific _____ to enter into the computer systems.

2. The _____ sheet is tubed at 11:00 A.M.

3. The N/O unit _____ the orders to the pharmacy.

4. The _____ devices are assigned to the staff by the health unit coordinator.

5. Lee feels that she is prepared to work the following day because she has taken _____.

6. The unit is assigned _____ tubes.

7. The password for the _____ allows the staff to make copies of information.

8. _____ information is not copied on the nursing unit.

9. Lee has agreed to work on the _____ unit the following day.

10. The communication book is used to share _____.

Multiple Choice Questions

1. Small-sized items that are used within a health care system may be sent through a _____ tube system.

   a. pneumatic

   b. yellow

   c. closed

   d. carrier

2. Items typically sent through an air-operated system include:

   a. Paper reports

   b. Medications

   c. Supplies

   d. All of the above

3. Copies of patient records may not be made without obtaining _____ permission from the patient.

   a. verbal

   b. written

   c. signed

   d. both b and c

4. Automatic dispensing machines are _____ storage devices or cabinets.

   a. laundry

   b. chart

   c. food

   d. drug

5. Most automated medication dispensing machines require a user _____ and identifier.

   a. password

   b. badge

   c. card

   d. none of the above

6. The advantage of an automated medication dispensing machine for a(n) _____ is that it allows drugs to be dispensed at the point of care.

   a. outpatient

   b. nurse

   c. physician

   d. inpatient

7. _____ are small mechanical pulley elevators that are used to transport supplies.

   a. Dumbwaiters

   b. Pneumatics

   c. Tubes

   d. None of the above

8. Items that can be transported by "dummies" include:

   a. Linen

   b. Tubing kits

   c. Dressings

   d. All of the above

9. A room call system allows _____ to communicate directly with the workstation via a two-way voice system.

   a. patients

   b. housekeeping

   c. physicians

   d. dietary

10. It is important to inform all patients how to use the _____ _____ system.

    a. emergency call

    b. recording chart

    c. rapid response

    d. IV start

CRITICAL THINKING EXERCISE

Unit-Specific Equipment

Visit a patient care unit, and make a list of all the different equipment you see. Ask the health unit coordinator to explain the use of each piece of equipment. Complete the chart below.

Equipment	What Is It Used For?	Ease of Use (Rate on a scale of 1 to 5, in which 1 is easy to use and 5 requires special training and passwords)
Telephone		
Fax machine		
Printer		

■ CASE SCENARIO ANSWERS

1. password
2. dietary
3. scans
4. VCS
5. notes
6. four
7. copier
8. Patient
9. N/O
10. information

■ MULTIPLE CHOICE ANSWERS WITH RATIONALES

1. **a.** *Pneumatic tubes* carry small-sized items through an air-operated system. (page 274)
2. **d.** Items typically sent through an air-operated system include *paper reports, medications, and supplies*. (page 274)
3. **d.** Copies of patient records cannot be made without first obtaining *written, signed* permission from the patient. (page 277)
4. **d.** Automated dispensing machines are *drug* storage devices or cabinets. (page 520)
5. **a.** Most automated medication dispensing machines require a user *password* and identifier. (page 520)
6. **d.** The advantage of an automated medication dispensing machine for an *inpatient* is that it allows drugs to be dispensed at the point of care. (page 520)
7. **a.** *Dumbwaiters* are small mechanical pulley elevators that are used to transport supplies. (page 73)
8. **d.** Items that can be transported by "dummies" include *linens, dressings, and tubing kits*. (page 73)
9. **a.** A room call system allows *patients* to communicate directly with the workstation via a two-way voice system. (page 275)
10. **a.** It is important to inform all patients how to use the *emergency call* system. (page 276)

SECTION 4

Professional Development

CHAPTER 16

Training

- ◆ Attend in-service training sessions.
- ◆ Attend department staff or health unit coordinator meetings.

Recommended Reading

Read and review Chapters 10 and 32 of *Health Unit Coordinator: 21st Century Professional.*

Abbreviations

CPOE   computerized physician order entry

Key Terms

Palliative care   comfort or end-of-life care

ꞔASE SCENARIO

Edna is a certified health unit coordinator with 15 years of experience. Tawanda is a new health unit coordinator who just started a few months ago. Although they differ in knowledge and experience, they both attend some of the same meetings and in-services. Every month they attend the staff meeting on their respective nursing units to discuss staff concerns and to hear about changes that their manager has been asked by the administration staff to share with them. Tawanda likes attending this meeting because all of the nurses and nursing assistants attend, as well as the health unit coordinators from the unit, and the outcome is better communication and cooperation among the staff.

They both attend monthly health unit coordinator meetings, at which information specific to health unit coordinators is provided. The information includes changes in health unit coordinator procedures, order entry, and ancillary department services. This meeting often includes guest speakers from the ancillary departments, because those departments realize the important role that health unit coordinators play in scheduling and preparing patients for exams to be completed in their departments. Edna and Tawanda especially look forward to the meetings that the dietary department attends, because dietary provides treats as a "thank you" for staff cooperation. Edna and Tawanda also attend a mandatory annual safety meeting for all employees in which infection control, body mechanics, fire safety, and disaster preparations are discussed. Edna has also attended meetings as the health unit coordinator representative on the committees that work on computer downtime process, unit communication with transporters, and quality improvement.

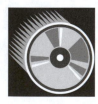

As a way to enhance her skills, Edna has attended continuing education classes during the past few years. Edna attended a class offered by the nursing education department entitled "The Dos and Don'ts of Preceptorship," which was designed for health unit coordinator and nursing assistant preceptors. Edna also attended a workshop on cancer and palliative care, "Oncology Seminar for Health Unit Coordinators," which was offered by the local chapter of National Association of Health Unit Coordinators (NAHUC). Last year, Edna went to the NAHUC annual education conference and attended sessions on computerized physician order entry (CPOE), ethnic diversity, and high-impact communication skills. This year, Edna has set a goal for herself that she will sit for the national health unit coordinator certification exam.

Case Scenario Questions

Indicate whether the following statements are true or false.

1. New employees as well as experienced employees need to attend annual infection control in-services.

2. Workshops offered by nursing education are only for nurses.

3. Only experienced health unit coordinators should attend the monthly health unit coordinator meetings.

4. New employees only need to attend meetings on body mechanics.

5. All employees need to attend fire safety meetings every month.

6. Disaster preparedness in-services need to be attended every year.

7. Noncertified health unit coordinators can attend workshops presented by local chapters of the NAHUC.

8. Nurses and nursing assistants only attend unit staff meetings.

9. Noncertified health unit coordinators can attend the NAHUC annual education conference.

10. Representatives from ancillary departments often attend monthly health unit coordinator meetings.

Multiple Choice Questions

1. Which of the following employees should attend health and safety training?

   a. All health care staff

   b. Health unit coordinators

   c. Maintenance employees

   d. Only nurses

2. Which of the following is a government department?

   a. Infection control department

   b. Risk management department

   c. Centers for Disease Control

   d. Joint Commission

3. Which of the following is an example of a mandatory meeting?

   a. Unit staff meeting

   b. Safety meetings

   c. Monthly health unit coordinator meeting

   d. Quality improvement meeting

4. Which of the following is a way to learn more about one's roles and responsibilities in the health care workplace?

   a. Work on committees

   b. Attend in-services

   c. Be a preceptor

   d. All of the above

5. What does the abbreviation PPE stand for?

   a. Personal protective equipment

   b. Professional protective equipment

   c. Para protective equipment

   d. Patient protective equipment

6. Attending which of the following constitutes continuing education?

   a. Body mechanics meetings

   b. Staff meetings

   c. NAHUC workshops

   d. Fire safety meetings

7. Health and safety committees monitor safety issues, including which of the following?

   a. Medication errors

   b. Patient falls

   c. Fire safety

   d. All of the above

8. Which employees should participate as health and safety committee members?

   a. Nurses

   b. Pharmacists

   c. Health unit coordinators

   d. A variety of health care team members

9. NAHUC offers educational opportunities via which of the following?

   a. Workshops

   b. Web site questionnaires

   c. A lending library

   d. All of the above

10. Which of the following answers best completes this sentence: A valuable employee seeks out new _____?

    a. Responsibilities

    b. Shortcuts

    c. Gossipers

    d. Ways of getting to work

CRITICAL THINKING EXERCISE

Professional Development

Use this worksheet to record answers to the following exercises.

1. Visit the NAHUC Web site at http://www.nahuc.org and determine where and when the next educational conference is being held.

   _____

   _____

   _____

   _____

   _____

2. Review the e-learning opportunities that are offered on the NAHUC Web site. List all five e-learning opportunities, print one out, and complete the quiz.

   _____

   _____

   _____

   _____

   _____

■ CASE SCENARIO ANSWERS

1. True
2. False
3. False
4. False
5. False
6. True
7. True
8. False
9. True
10. True

■ MULTIPLE CHOICE ANSWERS WITH RATIONALES

1. **a.** *All health care workers* need to attend annual health and training in-services. (page 149)
2. **c.** *Centers for Disease Control* is a government department. (page 146)
3. **b.** *Safety meetings* are mandatory meetings. (page 149)
4. **d.** *Working on committees, attending in-services,* and *precepting* are all ways to enhance your role and responsibilities. (page 594)
5. **a.** PPE is the abbreviation for *personal protective equipment.* (page 139)
6. **c.** A *workshop* is the best example of a continuing education offering. (page 594)
7. **d.** Health and safety committees monitor safety issues including *medication errors, patient falls,* and *fire safety.* (page 148)
8. **d.** *A variety of health care team members* or *a multidisciplinary staff* should participate in the health and safety committee. (page 148)
9. **d.** The NAHUC offers *workshops, Web site questionnaires,* and *a lending library* for continuing education opportunities. (page 594)
10. **a.** A valuable employee seeks out new *responsibilities.* (page 594)

■ CRITICAL THINKING EXERCISE ANSWERS

1. Multiple answers are possible, depending on when the site is accessed.
2. Health unit coordinator course, lending library, annual education conference, seminars/workshops, and completing the questionnaire in the *Coordinator.*

CHAPTER 17

Individual Development

◆ Review job-related publications (e.g., NAHUC Standards of Practice, journals, etc.).

◆ Review facility-specific publications, memos, policies, and so forth.

◆ Pursue and maintain certification.

Recommended Reading

Read and review Chapters 2, 11, and 32 of *Health Unit Coordinator: 21st Century Professional*.

Abbreviations

P&P   policy and procedures

Key Terms

Trade journal   a publication for a specific profession

CASE SCENARIO

Victor has been a certified health unit coordinator for eight years on the coronary critical care unit. Victor is very efficient at transcribing physician orders. He demonstrates excellent skill in his interpersonal interactions with staff and visitors. The staff members in Victor's department trust the work he does, and they depend on him to keep the department organized and running smoothly. The coronary care physicians rely on Victor to obtain current laboratory results and other reports. Victor realizes that he has an important role in his health care team, but sometimes he feels that he might not be viewed as a professional. Victor has expressed his feelings to his manager. Victor's manager does not want to lose Victor and wants to encourage him to develop professionally.

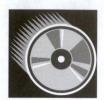

Case Scenario Questions

1. Imagine that you are Victor's manager, and you want to encourage him to develop two professional goals, one of which is obtaining national certification as a health unit coordinator. Write down your dialogue with Victor and the steps that you would suggest to him to pursue professional goals.

_____

_____

_____

_____

_____

_____

2. Imagine that you are Victor and write down your plan to achieve two professional goals, one of which is obtaining national certification as a health unit coordinator.

_____

_____

_____

_____

_____

_____

Multiple Choice Questions

1. National certification for health unit coordinators is awarded for what time period?
   a. 12 months
   b. 24 months
   c. 36 months
   d. 48 months

2. Certification can be defined as compliance with:
   a. A set of standards
   b. State regulatory laws
   c. The Patients' Bill of Rights
   d. A health unit coordinator job description

3. How many NAHUC contact hours are needed for each recertification cycle?
   a. 12
   b. 24
   c. 36
   d. 48

4. Which of the following statements best describes the NAHUC Standards of Practice?
   a. Statements that address professional conduct
   b. Standards that protect private health information
   c. An expression of where health unit coordinators want to be in the future
   d. Guidelines that can be used as a model of performance for health unit coordinators

5. Which of the following standards address confidentiality and are directed toward health care providers?
   a. DHHS
   b. HIPAA
   c. HICPAC
   d. PHI

6. What is the name of the National Association of Health Unit Coordinators' quarterly publication?
   a. NAHUC News
   b. The Coordinator
   c. The Reporter
   d. HUCs in the News

7. The health unit coordinator certification exam questions are based upon which of the following?
   a. A national job task analysis
   b. Joint Commission guidelines
   c. Health unit coordinator policy and procedures
   d. NAHUC Standards of Practice

8. Which of the following is not an option for recertification?
   a. Contact hours option
   b. Continuous employment option
   c. Certification exam option
   d. None of the above are recertification options

9. Whose responsibility is it to collect, save, and submit all documentation of recertification activities?
   a. The certified health unit coordinator's employer
   b. The certified health unit coordinator's manager
   c. The certified health unit coordinator
   d. The National Association of Health Unit Coordinators

10. Candidate handbooks for the certification exam can be obtained from:
    a. The National Association of Health Unit Coordinators' Web site
    b. The National Association of Health Unit Coordinators' office
    c. College and hospital bookstores
    d. Both a and b

CRITICAL THINKING EXERCISE

NAHUC Standards of Practice and Code of Ethics

Use the following tear-out worksheet for this activity. Visit the NAHUC Web site at http://www.nahuc.org or review pages 31–34 of *Health Unit Coordinator: 21st Century Professional* to complete this worksheet.

1. The NAHUC Standards of Practice are divided six main categories. List all six in order.

   a. _____

   b. _____

   c. _____

   d. _____

   e. _____

   f. _____

2. The NAHUC Code of Ethics is divided into five principles. List all five in order.

   a. _____

   b. _____

   c. _____

   d. _____

   e. _____

3. Explain one of the five principles of the NAHUC Code of Ethics in your own words.

   _____

   _____

   _____

   _____

   _____

4. Write about a personal example that demonstrates how you have already put one of the NAHUC Code of Ethics principles into practice, either as a student or an employee.

   _____

   _____

   _____

   _____

CRITICAL THINKING EXERCISE

Facility-Specific Publication, Memos, and Policies

Take this worksheet to your internship or work site and answer the following questions.

1. In what publication(s) would one check the spelling of a diagnostic procedure?

   _____

   _____

2. In what publication(s) would one find the generic name for a brand name medication?

   _____

   _____

3. In what publication(s) would one find the protocol for respiratory isolation?

   _____

   _____

4. In what publication(s) would one determine whether or not a nuclear medicine scan requires patient preparation?

   _____

   _____

5. In what publication(s) would one determine what type of vial is needed to collect blood for a culture?

   _____

   _____

6. In what publication(s) would one find the fire escape route?

   _____

   _____

7. In what publication(s) would one determine how to access a laboratory result from the information system?

   _____

   _____

■ CASE SCENARIO SUGGESTED ANSWERS

1. The manager may want to give Victor information on the National Association of Health Unit Coordinators and explain that the association's mission is to promote health unit coordinating as a profession through education and certification. The manager could encourage Victor to get involved with other people like himself in the association who want to develop professionally. The manager could encourage Victor to pursue certification. The manager could tell Victor how he or she would support Victor's goals.

2. Victor could choose to join a professional association and become certified as his goals. If he wants to join an association first, he could write a plan about how he would obtain a membership application, complete it, and return it. For his certification goal, he could give himself a time frame in which to prepare for the exam. He could make plans to obtain information about the exam content outline and study materials. He could also make plans to budget for the exam fee if his employer does not offer reimbursement.

■ MULTIPLE CHOICE ANSWERS WITH RATIONALES

1. **c.** National certification for health unit coordinators is awarded for *36 months*. (page 28)

2. **a.** Certification can be defined as compliance with *a set of standards*. (page 28)

3. **c.** One may recertify with *36 NAHUC contact hours* every three years. (page 30)

4. **d.** The NAHUC Standards of Practice are *guidelines that can be used as a model of performance for health unit coordinators*. (page 31)

5. **b.** *HIPAA* addresses confidentiality and is directed toward health care providers. (page 170)

6. **b.** The *Coordinator* is the name of the National Association of Health Unit Coordinators' quarterly publication. (page 14)

7. **a.** The health unit coordinator certification exam questions are based upon *a national job task analysis*. (page 590)

8. **b.** *Continuous employment* is not an option for recertification. (page 592)

9. **c.** It is the *certified health unit coordinator's* responsibility to collect, save, and submit all documentation of recertification activities. (page 592)

10. **d.** Candidate handbooks for the certification exam can be obtained from *the National Association of Health Unit Coordinators Web site* and *office*. (page 593)

REVIEW QUESTIONS

The following set of questions is a 50-item review that parallels the current content outline of the national certification exam. Thirty-five percent of the review questions fall under the category of transcription of orders, 47% are on the coordination of the health unit, 15% are on equipment and technical procedures, and 3% are on professional development.

1. Which of the following is the correct nonmilitary time for 2330 hours?
   a. 1:30 AM
   b. 3:30 AM
   c. 1:30 PM
   d. 11:30 PM

2. Staff members who work evening and night shifts on the same unit may get written unit staff information via the _____.
   a. phones
   b. answering machine
   c. bulletin boards
   d. call system

3. Which department focuses on ADLs?
   a. Physical therapy
   b. Occupational therapy
   c. Speech therapy
   d. Recreational therapy

4. TENS are ordered from which department?
   a. Central service
   b. Pharmacy
   c. Physical therapy
   d. Occupational therapy

5. In the order "1000 ml of D5W," *ml* stands for which of the following?
   a. Milliequivalent
   b. Milliliters
   c. Millimeter
   d. Mega liter

6. In the order "1000 ml of D5W @50cc/hr," *@50cc/hr* refers to the:
   a. Additives
   b. Amount
   c. Rate
   d. Solution

7. Which of the following is the correct meaning of QID?
   a. Every day
   b. Every other day
   c. Three times a day
   d. Four times a day

8. _____ can be used to generate orders, schedule procedures, and bill insurance companies.
   a. Beepers
   b. PCA
   c. Computers
   d. Faxes

9. The acronym NSAID stands for which of the following?

   a. Nonsteroidal anti-inflammatory drug

   b. Non sodium anti-inflammatory drug

   c. Non sublingual anti-inflammatory drug

   d. Non suspension anti-inflammatory drug

10. Which of the following is the correct spelling for the term that refers to comfort care orders?

    a. Palliative care

    b. Pallative care

    c. Pallitive care

    d. Pallaitive care

11. An OOB is an example of what type of order?

    a. Activity

    b. Observation

    c. Positioning

    d. Vital signs

12. Which of the following is the same as a consistent carbohydrate diet?

    a. Calorie control diet

    b. Diabetic diet

    c. Low cholesterol diet

    d. Low protein diet

13. Which of the following is the correct definition for the term *bolus*?

    a. A little at a time

    b. All at once

    c. To be given orally

    d. To be given intramuscularly

14. Which of the following is the process of measuring and transmitting heart activity during hospitalization?

    a. Cardiac catheterization

    b. Electrocardiogram

    c. Holter monitor

    d. Telemetry

15. Which of the following is the best reason to include a *reason for exam* when entering orders?

    a. To give guidance when performing exams

    b. To give guidance when performing exams and reading the exam results

    c. To ensure that the right exam gets done

    d. To ensure that the right exam gets done and the hospital receives reimbursement for the exam

16. The _____ system in a health care facility allows patients to communicate directly with the workstation via a two-way voice system.

    a. fax

    b. room call

    c. pneumatic

    d. copy

17. Which of the following is the correct term for a prepackaged sterile swab and culture medium in a tube?

    a. C & S

    b. Culture medium

    c. Culturette

    d. Cytology slide

18. Which of the following best defines O & P?

    a. Oral and passive

    b. Oral and positive

    c. Ova and platelets

    d. Ova and parasites

19. Which of the following best describes independent transcription?

    a. The health unit coordinator takes full accountability for the transcription process

    b. The nurse does not double-check the transcription of the health unit coordinator

    c. The nurse may still sign off that the orders were seen

    d. All of the above

20. Which of the following should be performed just before the health unit coordinator signs his or her name to a completed set of transcribed orders?

    a. Communicate the orders to the nurse

    b. Prioritize

    c. Reread and check all work for accuracy

    d. Record orders on the Kardex

21. The _____ is one of the most widely used communication devices.

    a. PDA

    b. computer

    c. telephone

    d. beeper

22. Which of the following abbreviations stands for "against medical advice"?

    a. AGMA

    b. AMLA

    c. AWOL

    d. AMA

23. It is important to answer incoming calls as soon as possible; often, calls can be processed in less than _____.

    a. 5 minutes

    b. 1 minute

    c. 10 minutes

    d. 10 seconds

24. When a caller chooses to leave a message, it is important to _____ the message back to the caller.

    a. send

    b. repeat

    c. hand

    d. fax

25. When contact is made with body fluids, the health unit coordinator must:

    a. Wear a mask and gloves

    b. Record an incident report

    c. Shower

    d. Observe standard precautions

26. In-services and workshops held at health care facilities are forms of _____ education.

    a. standard

    b. continuing

    c. college

    d. nonstandard

27. To gather information for the patient activity board, the health unit coordinator may:

    a. Read the hospital formulary

    b. Access a patient's records from a previous admission

    c. Refer to the patient acuity system

    d. Access information from a patient's Kardex

28. When a patient asks the health care provider to telephone test results directly to him or her at the patient's home phone number and not to leave a message, under which key area of the HIPAA privacy act is this covered?

    a. Access to medical records

    b. Notice of privacy practices

    c. Confidential communications

    d. Complaints

29. When answering the telephone, it is important to provide the caller with your name, title, and _____.

    a. phone number

    b. address

    c. location

    d. date

30. In order for communication to be successful, the _____ must receive the message.

    a. sender

    b. receiver

    c. manager

    d. none of the above

31. Examples of clerical supplies used by health unit coordinators include:

    a. Computers, telephones, and fax machines

    b. Patient charts, laboratory reports, and radiology reports

    c. Pens, tape, paper clips, and message pads

    d. Specimen cups, bandage tape, and dressings

32. A daily charge is a charge that is generated for _____ rented by the day.

    a. nourishments

    b. equipment

    c. nonreusable supplies

    d. vendors

33. Emergencies in health care facilities may be categorized as different types of:

    a. Stats

    b. Arrests

    c. Codes

    d. Protocols

34. What is the name of the document in which a patient legally appoints someone to make health care decisions in the event that he or she cannot decide for him- or herself?

    a. Durable power of attorney for health care

    b. Living will

    c. Power of attorney

    d. Living advance directive

35. Which of the following is used to record any event within the heath care facility that could result in injury or loss?

    a. MSDS sheet

    b. Incident report

    c. Safety committee report

    d. General safety rules

36. What chart form does the patient use to give voluntary permission for a procedure after the purpose, benefits, and risks have been explained?

    a. Informed consent

    b. Release of responsibility

    c. Permit for anesthesia

    d. Consent for disposal

37. Which of the following is an example of a training situation that a health unit coordinator would *not* be responsible for?

    a. Orienting a nurse to the nonclinical operations of the department

    b. Orienting a nurse to the operation of a blood glucose meter

    c. Orienting a physician to the information system to retrieve a laboratory result

    d. Training a long-time health unit coordinator who has transferred from another unit

38. A list of all of the patients and their room numbers within a unit is called a:

    a. Census

    b. Patient classification

    c. Formulary

    d. Patient catalog

39. A(n) _____ admission is an admission that has been planned in advance.

    a. outpatient

    b. direct

    c. unscheduled

    d. scheduled

40. _____ is a way to enhance your position within the profession.

    a. Certification

    b. Precepting

    c. Training

    d. All of the above

41. Which of the following would the health unit coordinator use to enter information to be used by the health care facility in determining staffing needs for the upcoming shift?
    a. Change of shift report
    b. Patient classification system
    c. Hospital formulary
    d. Request for FTE

42. Which staff person enters information into the registration program?
    a. Health unit coordinator
    b. Admitting clerk
    c. Emergency department clerk
    d. All of the above

43. What can the health unit coordinator do when forms fall out of a patient's chart because the chart ring binders won't close?
    a. Thin the chart according to facility policy
    b. Remove all outdated progress and graphic notes, and file them
    c. Label an empty chart binder with the patient's name and start a second binder
    d. Contact the medical records or health information department to file the outdated forms

44. Patient care after discharge will likely be provided by which of the following?
    a. Meals on wheels
    b. Social services
    c. Home health care
    d. Discharge planning

45. The process of containing and preventing the spread of germs that cause disease is:
    a. Isolation
    b. Nosocomial control
    c. Biohazard
    d. Epidemiology

46. Environmental services are notified of a discharge so they may perform which of the following tasks?
    a. Stop delivery of food trays and nourishments
    b. Prepare the patient room for the next patient
    c. Transport the patient safely to the environment outside the hospital
    d. Arrange care for the patient's home environment

47. What tool is used to record a patient being transported off of a unit?
    a. Sign in/out sheet
    b. Kardex
    c. Unit census
    d. Shift report sheet

48. Which of the following statements about laboratory reports is untrue?
    a. They may be paper reports
    b. They may be delivered to the patient's room
    c. They may be electronic reports
    d. They may be faxed to the patient's unit

49. What may be affixed to patient supplies to ensure that the patient is charged correctly?
    a. A purchase order
    b. A purchase requisition
    c. A sticker with the patient's name on it
    d. A sticker with an item code on it

50. The _____ function (button) on the telephone should be used whenever the receiver is not directly communicating with the sender.
    a. hold
    b. forward
    c. transfer
    d. reset

ANSWERS WITH RATIONALES

(The page numbers in parentheses correspond to the *Health Unit Coordinator: 21st Century Professional* textbook.)

1. **d.** 2330 hours is the military time for 11:30 PM. (page 513)

2. **c.** Members who work off shifts on the same unit may get written staff information via the bulletin boards. (page 278)

3. **b.** Occupational therapy works with patients to develop activities of daily living. (page 539)

4. **c.** TENS are ordered from physical therapy. (page 538)

5. **b.** The *ml* stands for milliliters. (page 522)

6. **c.** The phrase *@50cc/hr* is the rate of the intravenous order. (page 522)

7. **d.** QID stands for four times a day. (page 511)

8. **c.** Computers can be used to generate orders, schedule procedures, bill insurance companies, and communicate information. (page 273)

9. **a.** NSAID stands for nonsteroidial anti-inflammatory drug. (page 498)

10. **a.** Palliative is the correct spelling. (page 490)

11. **a.** An OOB is an activity. (page 484)

12. **b.** *Consistent carbohydrates* is a term that is sometimes used when ordering diabetic diets. (page 462)

13. **b.** *Bolus* means to give all of the fluid at once. (page 456)

14. **d.** *Telemetry* is a process of measuring and transmitting heart activity during hospitalization. (page 440)

15. **b.** The reason for the exam is used to give guidance when performing exams and reading the exam results. (page 439)

16. **b.** The room-call system allows patients to communicate directly with the workstation via a two-way voice system. (page 275)

17. **c.** A *culturette* is a prepackaged sterile swab and culture medium in a tube. (page 407)

18. **d.** O & P is the approved abbreviation for ova and parasites. (page 407)

19. **d.** *Independent transcription* is when the health unit coordinator takes full accountability for the transcription process and the nurse does not double-check the orders; however, the nurse still needs to see new orders written by the physician. (page 400)

20. **c.** Prioritizing orders should be the first step in the transcription order, followed by writing it on the Kardex. Not every order needs to be verbally communicated to the nurse. The health unit coordinator should double-check her work before signing her name to the completed set of orders. (page 398)

21. **c.** The telephone is one of the most widely used communication devices. (page 263)

22. **d.** AMA is the abbreviation for "against medical advice." (page 211)

23. **b.** Incoming calls can often be processed in less than one minute. (page 265)

24. **b.** When a caller would like to leave a message, it is important to repeat the message back to the caller to make sure that you heard the information correctly. (page 266)

25. **d.** When contact is made with body fluids, the health unit coordinator must observe standard precautions. (page 156)

26. **b.** Continuing education at health care facilities can be in the form of in-services and workshops. (page 594)

27. **d.** To gather information for the patient activity board, the health unit coordinator may access the information from the patient's Kardex, where information about scheduled tests and treatments is listed. (page 76)

28. **c.** When a patient asks the health care provider to telephone test results directly to him or her at the patient's home phone number and not to leave a message, this is covered under the confidential communications area of the HIPAA privacy act. (page 170)

29. **c.** When answering the telephone at the workstation, it is important to provide the caller with your name, title, and location. (page 264)

30. **b.** The receiver must receive the message from the sender for communication to take place. (page 249)

31. **b.** Clerical supplies used by health unit coordinators include writing instruments, tape, paper clips, and paper forms. Computers, telephones, and fax machines are examples of equipment. Charts and reports are part of the patient's record. The nursing staff would use the specimen cups, bandage tape, and dressings for patient care. (page 127)

32. **b.** Daily charges are charges that are generated daily for equipment rented by the patient. (page 131)

33. **c.** Emergencies in health care facilities are usually called *codes*. (page 151)

34. **a.** The durable power of attorney for health care is the means by which an individual appoints another person to make decisions about his or her health care should the individual be unable to do so. (page 178)

35. **b.** An incident report is used to record any event within the heath care facility that could result in injury or loss. (page 139)

36. **a.** Informed consent must be signed prior to surgery. (pages 552 and 553)

37. **b.** Health unit coordinators are responsible for a variety of nonclinical training practices, but they would not orient someone to clinical equipment. (page 283)

38. **a.** A list of all of the patients and their room numbers within a unit is called a *census*. (page 75)

39. **d.** A scheduled admission is one that is arranged prior to admission. (page 217)

40. **d.** Ways to enhance your position within the profession include: certification, continuing education, precepting, committee work, taking on additional responsibilities, and moving up the career ladder. (page 590)

41. **b.** Health care facilities use patient classification systems to determine acuity levels for staffing. (page 75)

42. **d.** All staff members whose job description requires entering information into the registration program may do so. These may include health unit coordinators, admitting clerks, and emergency department clerks. (page 214)

43. **a.** Each health care facility has a policy for pulling certain forms when a record has become too large to handle. (page 207)

44. **c.** Home health agencies provide care to patients in their homes. (page 239)

45. **a.** The process of containing and preventing the spread of germs that cause disease is *isolation*. (page 139)

46. **b.** Environmental services cleans the patient room after discharge. (page 239)

47. **a.** A sign in/out sheet is used to record information when a patient is transported off of the unit. (page 76)

48. **b.** Laboratory reports may be paper or electronic, and they may print at the workstation printer. (page 429)

49. **d.** Health care facilities may use a manual or computerized charge system that utilizes coded supply stickers. (page 129)

50. **a.** The hold button on the telephone should be used whenever the receiver is not directly communicating with the sender. (page 268)